Finance, Budgeting & Quantitative Analysis

A PRIMER FOR NURSING HOME ADMINISTRATORS

BRIAN GARAVAGLIA, PhD, FACHCA

HCPro

Finance, Budgeting & Quantitative Analysis: A Primer for Nursing Home Administrators is published by HCPro, Inc.

Copyright © 2013 HCPro, Inc.

Cover Image © Don Bishop. Used under license from Photodisc.

All rights reserved. Printed in the United States of America.   5 4 3 2 1

Download the additional materials of this book at *www.hcpro.com/downloads/11118*.

ISBN: 978-1-61569-196-8

No part of this publication may be reproduced, in any form or by any means, without prior written consent of HCPro, Inc., or the Copyright Clearance Center (978-750-8400). Please notify us immediately if you have received an unauthorized copy.

HCPro, Inc., provides information resources for the healthcare industry.

HCPro, Inc., is not affiliated in any way with The Joint Commission, which owns the JCAHO and Joint Commission trademarks.

Brian Garavaglia, PhD, FACHCA, Author
Melissa D'Amico, Associate Editor
James DeWolf, Editorial Director
Mike Mirabello, Graphic Artist
Matt Sharpe, Senior Manager of Production
Shane Katz, Art Director
Jean St. Pierre, Vice President of Operations and Customer Relations

Advice given is general. Readers should consult professional counsel for specific legal, ethical, or clinical questions.

Arrangements can be made for quantity discounts. For more information, contact:

HCPro, Inc.
75 Sylvan Street, Suite A-101
Danvers, MA 01923
Telephone: 800-650-6787 or 781-639-1872
Fax: 800-639-8511
Email: *customerservice@hcpro.com*

Visit HCPro online at:
www.hcpro.com and www.hcmarketplace.com

04/2013
22017

Table of Contents

A Word From the Author ix

Introduction xi

    Basic Principles of Financial Management in Long-Term Care xi

Chapter 1: The General Accounting Procedure 1

    The Accounting Equation 2

    Cash Accounting vs. Accrual Accounting 3

    Bookkeeping vs. Accounting 4

    Basic Financial Terminology 5

Chapter 2: Financial Statements 7

    The Income Statement 7

    The Balance Sheet 9

    The Cash Flow Statement 12

Chapter 3: The Financial Captain: The Balance Sheet 15

    Debits, Credits, and Postings to Accounts 17

    Accounting for Accruals and Deferrals 22

Chapter 4: The Accounting Cycle 23

    Closing Accounts 25

    Writing Off Uncollectible Accounts 27

TABLE OF CONTENTS

    Working Capital 29

    Net Operating Margin 30

    Current Ratio and Debt-to-Equity Ratio 31

    Capitalization Ratio 32

    Average Collection Period Ratio and Accounts Payable Average Payment Period Ratio 33

    Return on Assets and Return on Equity 35

    Other Useful Ratios 35

    Depreciation and Depreciation Expense 36

Chapter 5: Inventory 41

    Procedures for Handling Cash Funds 43

    Surety Bonds and the Conveyance of Funds 46

    Banking and Reconciliation 47

Chapter 6: Planning and Budgeting 49

    The Strategic Plan 49

    Tackling the Budget 49

    Forecasting Capital 54

Chapter 7: Cost Containment in Long-Term Care 55

    Types of Costs 55

Chapter 8: PPDs as the Benchmark for Measurement 59

    Determining PPD 59

    PPD and the Entire Facility 61

    Monitoring Costs Through Spend-Downs 62

Chapter 9: Labor Costs 63

    What to Look For 63

    Overtime and Pool Use 66

    Absenteeism 67

    Turnover 68

TABLE OF CONTENTS

Chapter 10: The Staff 71

The Dietary Department 71

The Housekeeping Department 72

The Laundry Department 73

The Maintenance Staff 75

Chapter 11: Medicaid, Medicare, and Third-Party Payment 77

Medicaid 77

The Start of a New Era 78

Medicare 79

Third-Party Payment 87

Chapter 12: The Financial Implications for Insurance Policies 89

Property Insurance 89

Liability Insurance 89

Workers' Compensation 90

Taxes 90

Chapter 13: Consolidated Billing, the Prospective Payment System, and the MDS 93

Consolidated Billing 93

MDS Drives All Billing 96

Off-Cycle Assessments 98

Administrator Involvement 98

A Maze of RUGs and Minutes 99

The Importance of Certification 100

The New Version—MDS 3.0 101

Chapter 14: Quantitative Analysis for Long-Term Care Administrators 105

Traditional Scientific Tenets 105

Research Examined 108

TABLE OF CONTENTS

Chapter 15: Common Quantitative Analytical Techniques for Healthcare Administration 111

Quantitative Methods 111

Visual Methods of Examining Data 113

Examining Dispersion: The Spread of Scores 119

Standard Deviation 120

Chapter 16: Correlation: The Importance of Measuring Relationships Between Variables 125

The Pearson Product Moment Correlation Coefficient 125

Chapter 17: Inferentially Based Statistical Procedures 131

Hypotheses 131

Additional Tests 134

ANOVA: A More Powerful Measuring Tool 137

Chapter 18: The Time Value of Money and Forecasting 143

Compounding and Discounting 143

Future Investments 144

Break-Even Analysis 146

Forecasting: Looking Into the Future 148

Using Regression Analysis as a Source of Forecasting 157

John Stuart Mill: The Logic Behind Causal Understanding 159

Chapter 19: Planning Through the Use of Networks 167

Program Evaluation Review Technique 167

Decision-Making in Long-Term Care 171

Programmed and Nonprogrammed Decisions 171

Conditions of Certainty, Uncertainty, and Risk 172

Chapter 20: Basic Economic Principles 177

Economic Resources and Economic Efficiency 178

What Is the Gross Domestic Product? 182

TABLE OF CONTENTS

Inflation, Unemployment, and Economic Growth 184

Supply and Demand in the Market Economy 186

Shifts in the Scale of Production 189

Consumer Behavior and Utility 191

How Income and Substitution Effects Influence Consumer Behavior 194

Price Elasticity of Supply and Demand 195

Marginal Analysis 196

Total Revenue and Costs and Marginal Revenue and Costs 198

References and Suggested Readings 201

> See page xiv for a complete list of the additional materials that accompany this book. Don't forget to check out the bonus chapter, "Mathematical Review," also included with these resources!

A Word From the Author

The current text, *Finance, Budgeting & Quantitative Analysis: A Primer for Nursing Home Administrators*, is an extension from a previous book that I wrote that was entitled *Finance and Budgeting for the Nursing Home Professional*. As was the case with the previous book, this book is written for professionals who do not have an extensive knowledge of financial or quantitative analysis. This book maintains many of the important financial concepts that were introduced by the previous text. However, this book expands on some areas and has added two important chapters: one highlighting healthcare economics as well as a chapter to refresh one's knowledge of some important mathematical concepts and to introduce some other mathematical concepts that can be used in managerial decision-making.

Financial and quantitative analysis is an important part of the daily mind-set of long-term care administrators, and yet finance and quantitative analysis are often the most daunting areas they address. Most individuals who oversee long-term care facilities are typically not financial specialists by training, and, as a result, dealing with large revenue and expenses creates a high level of anxiety and apprehension. Even though healthcare administrators address more than financial and quantitative matters, these skills often are closely aligned with other areas that they oversee. Therefore, administrators need to not only be conversant in financial and quantitative analysis, but they also have to feel fairly comfortable in using some important financial and quantitative skills to help make important managerial decisions.

This book provides a myriad of resources that the administrator frequently has to call upon in making daily decisions, although not all of the resources will be used daily. It also provides some important skills for those that do not have an extensive level of training in financial and quantitative analysis. Furthermore, it focuses on some skills that are specific to the healthcare industry—in particular nursing home care—such as using and determining per patient days as part of the daily budgeting process. Although this book will not turn readers into finance or quantitative analysis experts, it should help give nursing home administrators a sound understanding of the skills necessary for making important financial decisions that will impact the entire facility.

A WORD FROM THE AUTHOR

Upon completing this book, the reader should have a better understanding of what a balance sheet, income statement, statement of cash flow, and retained earnings statement are. Readers should also have a better understanding of how these four financial statements do not just exist in exclusivity but are intricately related to each other. Additionally, readers should have a better understanding of the importance of correctly posting to specifically identified accounts and how these accounts are closed. I hope that readers will leave this book with a sound understanding of some basic equations for calculating important financial ratios. Furthermore, readers should be able to have a better understanding of important budgeting skills, especially based on HPPDs and DPPDs. This book should also help to provide the administrator or prospective administrator with a rudimentary understanding of important macro- and microeconomic concepts that are involved in the larger realm of healthcare economics. Finally, readers will be able to refresh and even possibly enhance some important mathematical skills that can be used for further quantitative decisions they may encounter.

Although many will not need to rely on pencil and paper, since much of the financial and quantitative data analysis that is done in healthcare today is completed on the computer, administrators still need to understand the meaning of the financial and quantitative concepts as well as have a working knowledge of when and what type of financial and quantitative skills are needed to make sound and clear decisions. Today, managers have sophisticated financial and statistical programs that save many hours of laborious mathematical work in accounting, finance, and quantitative analysis. Yet, one still has to understand the meaning behind these important numbers.

This book helps to lead administrators through many of the procedures they can follow to obtain the answers they need to make the correct managerial decisions. It can be used as an important reference to look up areas that may assist the administrator, and it can provide the administrator with certain tools for data analysis and decision-making. Those that read this book should not feel that they have to memorize everything found in the forthcoming text. However, having the book available to them should make many administrators more comfortable, especially as a reference tool they can readily rely upon.

I would like to once again thank the people of HCPro, Inc., especially Ms. Adrienne Trivers, senior managing editor, and Ms. Melissa D'Amico, associate editor, who worked closely with me on this project. I would also like to thank the American College of Health Care Administrators, who helped to initially get Ms. Trivers and me together. I hope this new book will become an important and welcomed resource for many nursing home administrators.

Very truly yours,

Brian Garavaglia, PhD, FACHCA

Introduction

Basic Principles of Financial Management in Long-Term Care

Nursing home administrators do not have to be accountants or financial experts. However, they do need to have some basic knowledge of the accounting and financial process. This will help them to understand important financial statements, as well as be able to pose informed questions to other experts, such as the accountant(s) who usually compile the financial reports for the nursing facility. It is important to understand that although the administrator may not be an accountant by training, he or she ultimately holds the position of chief financial officer for the facility. This is why it is so imperative that administrators have a basic understanding of important financial principles that will help them to make informed decisions.

As noted in the preceding paragraph, most facilities now use accountants who are employed either within a larger corporate structure or contractually to perform accounting and financial analysis. This helps to relieve the administrator from having to compile accounting and financial reports, which is time-consuming and must be addressed by a professional who maintains strict compliance with the Generally Accepted Accounting Principles (GAAP), the standard framework of guidelines for financial accounting (more on this later). Also, due to the myriad new tax laws that are generated each year, specific forms that need to be used, and the complexity of cost accounting, especially as it relates to Medicare and Medicaid rules, an accountant who specializes in long-term financial information is an important asset to a facility. The administrator has enough to deal with, what with maintaining compliance to specific state and federal regulations, handling staff issues, addressing project development and plant operation issues, setting specific budgets, and developing marketing plans, among other tasks, without having to also worry about creating accounting and financial reports for the facility.

INTRODUCTION

This is not to say that administrators are totally hands-off in this area. Usually the administrator handles much of the internal accounting. This can include such tasks as establishing budgets; calculating monthly Medicare revenue; completing trust fund auditing; interest allocation and reconciliation; documenting revenue recognized from Medicare, private pay, hospice, and other sources; reconciling bank statements; calculating payables, including payroll and payroll taxes; examining and reconciling bills and their respective costs; examining aging reports; and calculating average cost per resident day to determine how efficiently the facility is using its resources. The administrator often compiles and analyzes this data and submits his or her analysis to the facility accountant(s) so that they can complete their important work. Therefore, the administrator is the point person who obtains the necessary information, performs his or her internal financial analysis, sends it to the accountant(s) as important source documentation so that they can complete their work, and eventually receives from the accountant(s) the larger picture of all this financial information in the form of financial reports, including income statements, balance sheets, and cash flow reports, among others.

DOWNLOAD YOUR MATERIALS NOW

Readers of *Finance, Budgeting & Quantitative Analysis: A Primer for Nursing Home Administrators* can download the following items by visiting the HCPro Web address below. Electronic file names in parentheses correspond with the following documents. We hope you will find these downloads useful:

- **(D1)** Explanation of the Present Value Factor of $1, Future Value Factor of $1, and the Normal Distribution Chart
- **(D2)** Future Value of $1 Spreadsheet
- **(D3)** Income Statement, Balance Sheet, Statement of Retained Earnings, and Cash Flow Statement
- **(D4)** Inter-committee Action Request
- **(D5)** Medicare Reconsideration Request Form
- **(D6)** Medicare Redetermination Request Form
- **(D7)** Meeting Attendance Record
- **(D8)** Meeting Checklist
- **(D9)** Meeting Minutes
- **(D10)** Normal Distribution Chart
- **(D11)** New Manager Skills Assessment
- **(D12)** Notice of Denial of Medical Coverage
- **(D13)** Notice of Denial of Payment
- **(D14)** Notice of Exclusion from Medicare Benefits
- **(D15)** Patient's Request for Medical Payment
- **(D16)** Patient Request for Medicare Payment (Spanish Version)
- **(D17)** Performance Review
- **(D18)** Present Value of $1 Spreadsheet
- **(D19)** Professional Development Form
- **(D20)** Request for a Medicare Hearing
- **(D21)** Skilled Nursing Facility Advanced Beneficiary Notice
- **(D22)** Transfer of Appeal Rights
- **BONUS CHAPTER:** Mathematical Review

www.hcpro.com/downloads/11118

Thank you for purchasing this product!

HCPro

1 The General Accounting Procedure

As I mentioned in the introduction, most, if not all, major financial reports must adhere to the Generally Accepted Accounting Principles (GAAP). The Financial Accounting Standards Board established the GAAP to provide uniformity among accounting professionals. The following are some of the major principles that are part of the GAAP standards:

1. **Objectivity:** Accounting is based on documenting factual and empirically based information. Some things, such as goodwill and the organization's reputation, are more difficult to account for, but, overall, important source documents, such as receipts, invoices, checks, documented cash transactions, and the like, comprise the objective information that accountants use to compile their financial reports.

2. **Conservatism:** Accountants are taught to be conservative. They always examine financial information with some level of skepticism. If there is doubt in their financial data, they choose the more conservative estimate. That means they choose the lesser of the two estimates for gains and the greater of the two estimates for losses, instead of maximizing gains and minimizing losses. If an accountant is wrong due to his or her conservatism, the accountant at least knows he or she is wrong because he or she underestimated the gains or overestimated the losses.

3. **Consistency:** The business entity—in this case, the long-term care facility—should use the same accounting procedure from one period to the next.

4. **The monetary principle:** Money is the key source of accounting measurement. This does not mean money just as observable cash but rather revenue or expenses that ultimately lead to cash-based transactions.

CHAPTER 1

5. **The accounting period:** This is usually a consistent time period, generally one year in duration. This is typically established as the organization's fiscal year.

6. **The full-disclosure principle:** The material in the financial statement should be accurate and be documented in an informative manner, such that someone who knows how to read a financial report can obtain an accurate picture of the facility's financial health. Therefore, ultimately all important financial information is included in the financial statement to present an accurate depiction of the financial entity that is not misleading.

7. **The matching principle:** This is the central feature in the double-entry accounting system established under GAAP. Revenue earned is matched against expenses accrued. When a debit entry exists, there is a corresponding credit entry.

The Accounting Equation

The matching principle mentioned in the preceding section gives way to the double-entry accounting principle. Balance is an important issue in accounting. What is taken from one area must be accounted for in another area. To better understand this, let's examine some basic elements in what is known as the accounting equation. The following is one view of the equation:

> **Assets = Equities**

Assets are all the tangible and intangible elements the nursing facility owns; this includes the building, the equipment, and even such things as goodwill. Equity is resources that are used to help purchase assets and investments. As you can see, assets equal equity. You can expand the equation even further to include not only assets and equity but also liabilities. Liabilities are the rights that creditors have against the business and are represented as debts of the nursing facility. Taking liabilities into consideration, the following equation results:

> **Assets = Liabilities + Owner's Equity**

Again, both sides of the equation balance equally. The total assets for the facility are equal to the total liabilities plus the owner's total equity in the healthcare facility. Another way to look at this is to put it

THE GENERAL ACCOUNTING PROCEDURE

into concrete numbers. Let's say a facility had in its balance sheet $10 million in assets. The balance sheet also reported $8 million in liabilities and $2 million in owner's equity. We can see that the $10 million in assets is equal to the $10 million in liabilities plus owner's equity.

We can expand the accounting equation one step further. Owners often want to know what their equity is in the business, regardless of whether the business is a sole proprietorship, a partnership, or a corporation with shareholders. The following equation demonstrates this:

> **Assets − Liabilities = Owner's Equity**

Given that assets are the tangible or intangible elements owned by the facility or organization, minus liabilities or the debts or rights of creditors against the business, what is left is the owner's equity. Because creditors have preferential rights to the assets of the business entity, the residual component subsequently left is owner's equity. Subsequently, reducing liability will help to enhance owner's equity.

Cash Accounting vs. Accrual Accounting

Businesses can use one of two basic systems of accounting: the cash accounting method or the accrual accounting method. When a business uses the cash accounting method, revenue is reported only when cash is received, and expenses are noted only when cash is disbursed. Small businesses may use this method, but most large businesses and most healthcare facilities use the accrual method. Most laws, federal and state auditors, as well as accountants employed by healthcare facilities and trained to engage in the accounting process through strict adherence to GAAP dictate use of the accrual method. The accrual accounting process reports revenue during the period in which it was earned and reports expenses during the period in which they were incurred. The following chart provides examples of both procedures:

Cash Basis	Accrual Basis
Revenue for January service received in February and noted in the books for February	Revenue for January service noted in the books for January, even though cash transaction was not received until February
Paid vendor $1,000 in February and noted in the books for February for supplies bought in January	Supplies costing $1,000 bought in January and noted as an expense on the January books even though bill was paid in February

CHAPTER 1

The accrual system of accounting is one of the fundamental features of modern accounting and the accounting profession. It further helps to standardize the accounting system, recognizing revenue and expenses at the time they are achieved or realized.

In healthcare facilities as well as other types of businesses, bills are often not paid exactly at the time they are realized. This applies not only for services the facility provides but also for expenses the facility must pay to those that help support its services. For example, you may have residents who do not pay their bill until the month after services are rendered (e.g., they pay in April for services they received in March); likewise, you may have residents who do not pay for their March and April services until May. Furthermore, the amount paid in each month may vary depending on the type of services rendered. As a final example, you may buy supplies in May—an expense to your facility—but you may have 60 days to pay the vendor from which you made the purchase.

As you can see, with the cash method it becomes somewhat unwieldy to determine when an actual revenue or expense was truly realized because this determination is based on when the actual cash transaction happened.

With the accrual method, you document that services were rendered in specific months for a specific amount and that an expense was realized for a specific amount during a specific month, regardless of when the cash was received or disbursed. This creates an objective and structured manner for determining monthly revenue and expenses. Usually, businesses, including healthcare facilities, use the month as the specific period during which the accrual system of accounting determines when revenue and expenses are realized. In other words, even though a cash payment was received in April and the facility paid cash in April for supplies it received, the cash received may have been for services rendered in March, which would be the month to which the revenue would be applied, and the cash disbursed may also be for a supplies expense for March and would be noted in the books as a disbursement for a March expense.

Bookkeeping vs. Accounting

Acute care facilities often deal with large and sophisticated billing and accounting procedures, and therefore they often need a few full-time accountants on staff. Accountants analyze financial information to help the facility make informative business decisions. Accounting is usually conducted by those who are specially trained in the area, with an emphasis toward compiling data to provide informative financial information regarding the business.

THE GENERAL ACCOUNTING PROCEDURE

Most nursing care facilities, assisted living facilities, and other types of sub-acute care facilities usually do not have an accountant employed internally, even though they have myriad accounting information that they need to address on a daily basis. This is where a bookkeeper plays a key role. A bookkeeper is usually employed internally in most long-term care environments. Typically, the bookkeeper—who is often not formally trained in accounting—handles many of the important entries that are eventually passed on to the facility's accountant. Bookkeepers address accounts receivable and accounts payable, entering receivables and payables when they are received or paid out; monitor patient billing; mail monthly statements to residents or their families; write checks; keep track of disbursements as they go out for payment on specific accounts; and make sure the office finances are being addressed in a timely and orderly fashion.

As you can see, the bookkeeper does most of the daily financial footwork. Hence, the bookkeeper holds an essential position in the long-term care environment. Even though most long-term care facilities employ external billing and accounting professionals to address most Medicare and Medicaid billing and copayments, their staff bookkeeper and administrator still must be aware of basic billing information regarding Medicare and Medicaid, as well as know where, when, and who should be contacted for specific copayments that are an important source of the healthcare landscape. Frequently, the administrator and the bookkeeper work together to compile the necessary internal financial information required to close out the books each month. This information is then submitted to the accounting and billing professionals at the end of the month.

Why employ an accountant and/or billing professional(s)?

Today, due to the labyrinth of special forms and paperwork that need to be filled out for Medicare and Medicaid reimbursement, facilities have called upon financial specialists who deal exclusively with the regulations and procedures inherent in Medicare and Medicaid reimbursement. The rules and regulations that govern this area need to be followed assiduously. If a simple protocol is not followed, or if it has changed and now prevents someone from following the appropriate procedure, it can prevent a facility from obtaining its revenue in a timely manner. And those who have worked within long-term care facilities understand that most facilities have a fixed budget and require timely remuneration. Because of this, it often makes sense for such facilities to hire financial professionals who exclusively address this area and are well informed regarding the rules and regulations that must be followed.

Basic Financial Terminology

Most healthcare managers are not accountants. However, whether you are an administrator within a nursing care facility, an assisted living facility, a sub-acute care facility, or even a hospital, you must have

CHAPTER 1

some basic understanding of financial information. I already mentioned some general terms, such as assets, liabilities, and equity. The following list defines these terms again, as well as presents some new terms:

1. **Assets:** These are the tangible or intangible elements a business owns, such as supplies, beds, and possibly such things as the reputation of the facility.

2. **Liabilities:** These are the facility's debts, or the claim that creditors have against the facility. This is why unpaid debts can lead to a creditor instituting a lien against the facility.

3. **Equity:** This can also comprise liabilities, because liabilities are a type of equity of the creditor's claim on that business until payment is complete. However, more specifically, it is the concern of owner's equity or shareholder's equity, in which owners or shareholders provide resources so that they have a claim on the business.

4. **Capital:** This is money invested in the facility. In addition, a facility's equipment and its employees are considered its capital.

5. **Revenue:** These are earnings garnered for providing specific healthcare services. Simply put, this is the money that is coming into the facility.

6. **Expenses:** This is the cost the facility accrues through rendering healthcare services. Again, simply put, this is what is going out of the facility to provide payment to vendors, supply companies, the staff, and so forth.

2 Financial Statements

Although accountants use numerous types of financial statements, the two most important for a healthcare administrator, especially in long-term care, are the income statement and the balance sheet. Often, a considerable amount of work goes into creating these financial statements, but once an administrator has these statements in front of him or her, they provide a substantial amount of information to help aid in business decisions. They also provide information that lends itself to further financial analysis by enabling administrators to determine such things as the facility's current working capital, quick ratio, and debt to equity. We will examine these types of analyses later in this chapter.

The Income Statement

The *income statement*, sometimes called the **profit and loss statement**, summarizes the revenue, expenses, and net income or loss of a business for a specific period, usually one month. Owners and administrators are often interested in knowing what their facility's net income or profit is, as well as possibly any loss incurred, for a particular month. The income statement helps to answer those questions. Generally speaking, net income is the excess of revenue over expenses, and net loss is the excess of expenses over revenue.

Paying close attention to the income statement from one month to another is important. Not only does it help to demonstrate the facility's financial activity over a specific period, but comparing the income statement from one month to the next helps to show any possible changes in revenue and/or expenses that may enhance or impair business operations. The following is an example of a very simple income statement:

CHAPTER 2

FIGURE 2.1
INCOME STATEMENT FOR XYZ NURSING HOME

March 2012

Revenue

Operating Revenue

Physical Therapy:	$ 40,000
Occupational Therapy:	$ 30,000
Speech Therapy:	$ 20,000
Medicaid:	$ 250,000

Nonoperating Revenue

Family Meals:	$ 1,000
Fundraiser:	$ 3,000

Total Revenue:	$ 344,000

Expenses

Operating Expenses

Salaries (total):	$ 225,000
Medical Supplies:	$ 10,000
Furniture:	$ 5,000
Medical Equipment:	$ 20,000
Utilities:	$ 1,000
Pharmacy:	$ 2,000
Kitchen Expansion:	$ 20,000

Nonoperating Expenses

Landscape Consultation:	$ 1,000

Total Expenses:	$ 284,000

Net Profit (Loss): $ 60,000

Taxes:	$ 40,000

Net Income (After Interest and Taxes): $ 20,000

FINANCIAL STATEMENTS

Although the preceding income statement is simplistic (in reality, healthcare facilities must account for far more types of revenue and expenses), it does demonstrate the basic concept of how an income statement is set up. Also, note in the example that net profit is not the same as net income. *Net profit* is equal to revenue minus expenses or earnings before interest and taxes (EBIT). However, the real bottom line is *net income*, or what's left after any interest and taxes are paid. (Often, these terms are used interchangeably, but for this example I used the preceding distinction to refer to the differences between the two concepts.) Finally, notice that revenue and expenses are often further divided into operating revenue and expenses, which are accrued or incurred as part of normal business operations, and nonoperating revenue and expenses, which are not usually part of normal business operations.

The Balance Sheet

The *balance sheet* is the second important financial statement that business entities often use when making financial decisions. Whereas the income statement examines a facility's financial activity over a specific period, the balance sheet examines its assets, liabilities, and owner's or shareholder's equity at a specific date. And whereas the income statement answers questions regarding how the facility performed financially during this time, the balance sheet answers questions such as what the facility has today or had on some other date.

To further clarify the distinction, the income statement examines the financial activity that occurs for a particular month, whereas the balance sheet informs the administrator of the company's financial status on a certain date. The balance sheet also helps to demonstrate how much cash, accounts receivable and payable, inventory, and owner's equity, among other things, exist on a specific date. In addition, the balance sheet is based on balancing: The assets on the balance sheet equal the liabilities plus the owner's equity. The following is an example of a simple balance sheet:

CHAPTER 2

FIGURE 2.2
BALANCE SHEET FOR XYZ NURSING HOME

April 30, 2012

Current Assets		Current Liabilities	
Cash:	$ 25,000	Accts. Payable:	$ 1,500,000
Accts. Rec.:	$ 100,000	Notes Payable:	$ 250,000
Inventory:	$ 25,000	Benefits:	$ 25,000
Prepaid Ins.:	$ 10,000		
Gov't. Securities:	$ 100,000		
Long-Term Assets		**Long-Term Liabilities**	
Land/Plant:	$ 5,000,000	Bonds Payable:	$ 1,500,000
Equipment:	$ 1,500,000	Mortgage Payable:	$ 3,500,000
Other Assets			
Goodwill/Intangible:	$ 300,000	**Total Liabilities:**	$ 6,775,000
Total Assets:	$ 7,060,000	**Owner's Equity**	
		Capital Stock:	$ 200,000
		Retained Earnings:	$ 85,000
		Total Liabilities and Net Worth:	$ 7,060,000

Although this is not an elaborate balance sheet, it does provide some important information. First, it shows that the total assets balance with the total liabilities plus net worth. Second, it shows us where the business stood financially when this balance sheet was completed. Third, it differentiates between current assets (those that will be converted to cash or received within a short period, usually one year or less) and long-term assets (those that extend beyond one year in duration). Fourth, it differentiates between current liabilities (those that must be paid within a short period, usually less than one year) and long-term liabilities (those that will be paid over a longer period). Finally, notice that the last part of the balance sheet examines the owner's equity. This is important because not only does it provide information regarding the business' capital, but it also leads to another important financial statement: the *statement of retained earnings*, which is often asked for as an important summary for tax purposes.

FINANCIAL STATEMENTS

To understand retained earnings, let's look at a simple example. John Doe owns the XYZ Nursing Home. His retained earnings were $150,000 on January 1, 2012. Given an owner's equity of $285,000, including capital stock with possible dividends, we will construct a statement of retained earnings for the XYZ Nursing Home. Also, instead of the balance sheet reflecting April 30, we'll change the fictional date to reflect December 31. The statement of retained earnings would look something like this:

FIGURE 2.3
STATEMENT OF RETAINED EARNINGS FOR XYZ NURSING HOME FOR YEAR ENDING DECEMBER 2012

John Doe, Capital Balance from Preceding Year:	$ 150,000
Add Net Income for 2012:	$ 85,000
Total Retained Earnings:	$ 235,000
Minus Paid Dividends:	($ 10,000)
Total Retained Earnings for 2012:	$ 225,000

Moving back to the balance sheet for a minute, James Gill, author of *Financial Analysis—The Next Step*, makes the distinction between a *safe corporation* and a *risk corporation*. He states that a safe corporation demonstrates "a low return, a large equity base, and slow growth with little debt and short-term assets." Conversely, he states that a risk corporation demonstrates "a high yield, high long-term assets, outside funds supporting over half of the business, a small equity base, fast growth, and large earnings fluctuations."

Let's examine what this means. A risk corporation demonstrates some important features. The following are the more glaring ones:

1. **High long-term assets:** You might think this is good, but numerous long-term assets can equal reduced liquidity, leading to a reduced amount that one can allocate to pay off one's current bills

2. **A large amount of outside funds supporting the business:** This means the business is highly leveraged and that many outside individuals, due to unpaid bills, have a legal claim on the business

3. **Small equity base:** This leads to less equity available to place into the business, and it does not make owners happy when their net worth in the company is reduced

CHAPTER 2

Conversely, a safe company has more assets tied up as part of its current assets and, therefore, has greater liquidity. Debt is reduced, especially long-term debt, allowing more funds to be allocated to deal with current liabilities. And finally, a larger equity base helps to support further capital expenditures that will potentially lead to an increase in assets, as well as increasing the net worth for the owner(s).

So, in regard to these terms, our example of the balance sheet for XYZ Nursing Home shows that the facility's total assets are divided as follows: current assets equal about 3.68%, long-term assets equal about 92.07%, and other assets equal 4.25%. Short-term liabilities make up 25.14%, long-term assets make up 70.82%, and owner's equity equals 4.04%. In short, this company would fit the criteria for a risk company. Its current assets are low, and its liquidity, especially in terms of meeting its short-term financial obligations, appears problematic. This is compounded by a significantly large amount of long-term assets and a large amount of long-term liabilities that will be plaguing the company for years to come. Finally, the owner's equity is low, impairing the ability to add additional capital to the company and not making owners very happy with the low level of net worth.

Facility comparisons

Another important piece of advice is to know how your company compares to others in your industry, to give you a better understanding of your company's financial position. For example, your balance sheet may appear poor when compared to that of a large auto parts company or even an assisted living facility. However, these are all different industries. Even in the healthcare industry, your balance sheet and the balance sheet of a hospital or assisted living facility may be dramatically different. In reality, hospitals, nursing facilities, sub-acute rehabilitation facilities, and even assisted living facilities are separate industries. Furthermore, geographic location plays an important role in financial analysis. Nursing facilities within large urban areas will often demonstrate a different financial disposition than those found in suburban and rural areas. Finally, other features, such as tax status and ownership type—for example, whether the facility is a nonprofit, for-profit, or state- or county-owned facility—also may play a role in financial analysis. In short, you cannot compare apples and oranges. Therefore, it is important that you know your industry standards and compare them to your financial analysis.

The Cash Flow Statement

Although the income statement and balance sheet are the bread-and-butter financial statements for the healthcare administrator, the cash flow statement is also important for healthcare administrators in long-term care facilities to be aware of when making important financial decisions.

FINANCIAL STATEMENTS

The *cash flow statement* is just that—a financial statement that examines the flow of cash from three major areas: operations, investing, and financing. It helps to demonstrate whether the cash that is being generated is adequate to support the business' current and future needs. The following is an example of a cash flow statement for XYZ Nursing Home:

FIGURE 2.4
CASH FLOW STATEMENT FOR XYZ NURSING HOME

December 31, 2012

Cash Received from Operating Activities:

Add

Cash received for Patient Services	$ 1,500,000	
Cash received from other medical services	$ 300,000	$ 1,800,000

(Minus)

Cash for payment of worker expenses		(1,500,000)

Net cash flow for operating activities: $ 300,000

Cash flows from investing activity:

Increased Cash Outlays for
    Medical Equipment: (25,000)

Increased Cash Outlays for
    Plant/building Updates/additions: ($ 250,000)

Net cash flow from investing activities ($ 275,000)

Cash flows from financing activities:

Issuance of capital stock:	$ 10,000	
Dividends Paid Out:	($ 5,000)	

Net cash flow from financing activities $ 5,000

Net increase/decrease in cash $ 30,000
Cash balance December 1, 2012 $ 195,000
Total cash $ 225,000

CHAPTER 2

Notice that in the previously described cash flow statement, cash flow from operating activity generated a net positive cash flow of $300,000. Conversely, cash flow from investing activities generated a net negative cash flow of $275,000. Finally, the net cash flow generated from financing activities was $5,000. Therefore, for the month of December, the XYZ Nursing Home generated a net cash flow of positive $30,000. The cash flow of $30,000 for the month of December is then added to the positive cash flow of $195,000 that the nursing home started the month of December with, resulting in $225,000 total cash. For the nursing home in this example, this outcome is not too bad but not great by any means. It is not out of the ordinary for facilities to have negative cash flow, which is a common problem often found in many healthcare facilities, including nursing homes.

Although the numbers are fictitious and do not bear any resemblance to those relating to most long-term care environments, this example demonstrates how cash flow statements work. Also, note that the "Operations" section—not reflected in this example—typically has most of the cash flow entries, especially for most nursing and other long-term care facilities. This is because in long-term care facilities, operational cash flow is the more prominent activity when compared to the activity found within the investing and financing areas. This is typical of most long-term care facilities. For instance, a long-term care facility generally invests less in equipment than, say, an acute care hospital would, especially in terms of investments in high-tech medical equipment, such as CAT scanners and MRI machines.

Also, it's important to note that financing for long-term care facilities can be variable. For instance, long-term care facilities that are under a large corporate umbrella would have a greater level of financial activity than that shown in our example of XYZ Nursing Home's cash flow statement. And the cash flow statement of an acute care facility usually would reflect even larger levels of financial activity, primarily due to the greater level of capital such a facility can devote to financing, something that is more limited in long-term care facilities and corporations.

3 The Financial Captain: The Balance Sheet

The previous chapter highlights a number of different financial statements, including the balance sheet, the income statement, the statement of cash flow, and the retained earnings statement. Although all these statements are important, the one that healthcare administrators often pay the most attention to when analyzing monthly financial activity is the income statement. This is because it provides administrators with a look at the financial activity over a period of time—usually 30 or 31 days. In reality, however, it is the balance sheet that is the "captain" of the financial statements. The balance sheet is where all of the financial data ultimately end up, and it provides an organization's financial status at a given period of time. Furthermore, the final totals found in the income statement, statement of retained earnings, and cash flow statement are all recorded in the balance sheet. Although administrators will not usually calculate and post this information—it is usually done by the facility's or organization's accountants—it is important to have a basic understanding of the balance sheet and how it interacts with other financial statements.

The following diagram illustrates the interaction between the balance sheet, the statement of cash flow, and the statement of retained earnings.

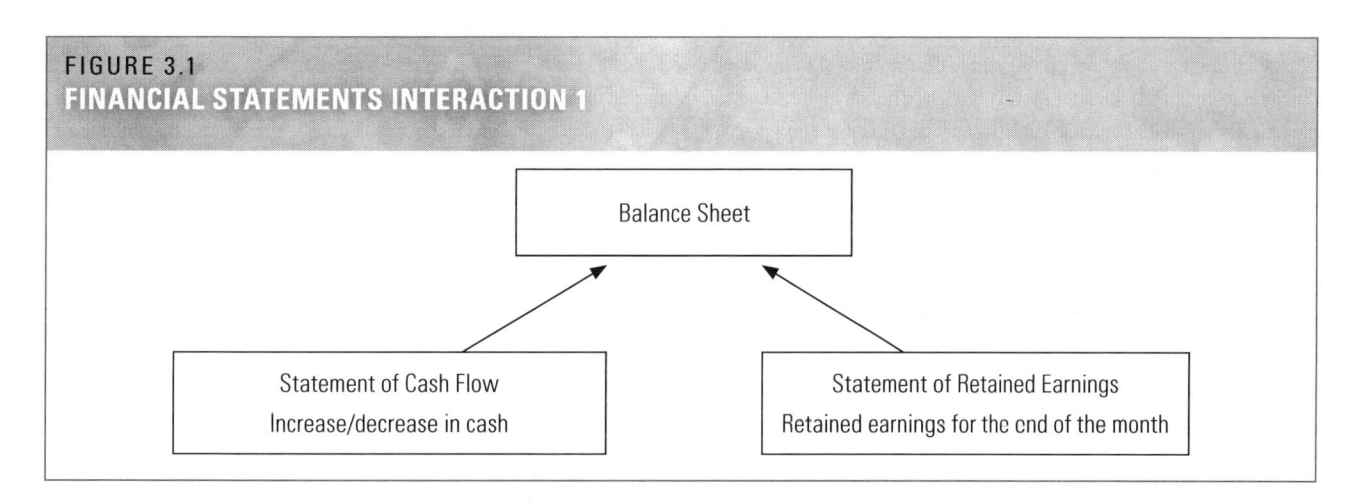

FIGURE 3.1
FINANCIAL STATEMENTS INTERACTION 1

Balance Sheet

Statement of Cash Flow
Increase/decrease in cash

Statement of Retained Earnings
Retained earnings for the end of the month

CHAPTER 3

First, notice that the statement of cash flow measures the movement of cash during a specific period, usually one month. The net cash flow for a specific month, regardless of whether it is positive or negative, is posted on current assets in the balance sheet. (More specifically, it can be posted under "Cash" in the assets section of the balance sheet.)

The statement of retained earnings documents the net income after any dividends have been paid out—this is the facility's retained earnings for the month. These retained earnings go back into the company and are posted in the balance sheet as well. This information can be found in the final part of the balance sheet, often referred to as stockholder's, shareholder's, or owner's equity.

These separate financial statements are never truly separate but work in close association. Again, it is important for the administrator to not only have some basic understanding of each of these financial tools but to also know how these tools work together.

To further enhance the interaction found between the different financial statements, the income statement has been added in the following example to demonstrate how this tool interacts with the statement of retained earnings and the balance sheet.

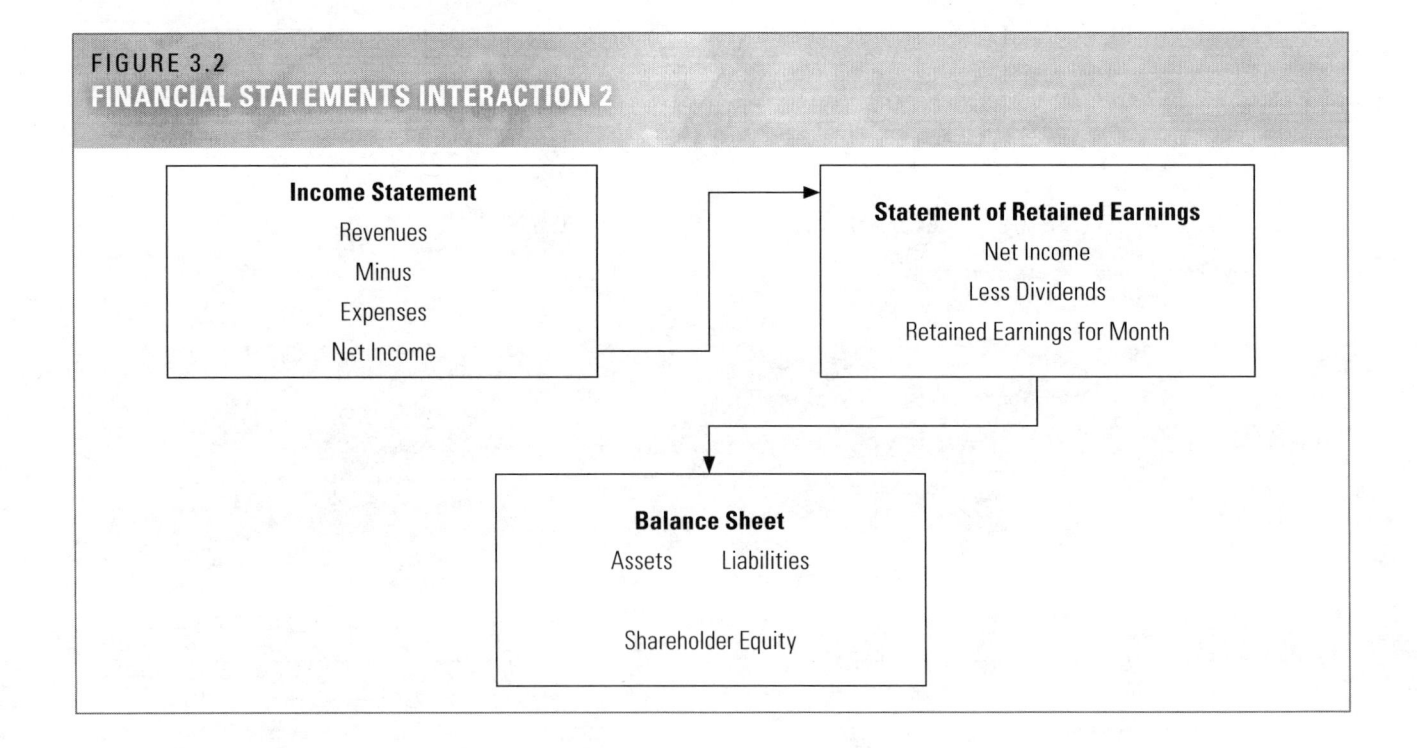

FIGURE 3.2
FINANCIAL STATEMENTS INTERACTION 2

Income Statement
Revenues
Minus
Expenses
Net Income

Statement of Retained Earnings
Net Income
Less Dividends
Retained Earnings for Month

Balance Sheet
Assets   Liabilities

Shareholder Equity

THE FINANCIAL CAPTAIN: THE BALANCE SHEET

The income statement examines the financial activity of an organization over a specific period of time, usually one month. The net income documented in the financial statement is transferred to the statement of retained earnings. The statement of retained earnings, minus any dividends paid out, leaves the facility with either a positive or negative net retained earnings for the month. The net retained earnings is then posted to the shareholder's equity section of the balance sheet.

Debits, Credits, and Postings to Accounts

Many people have a mistaken impression of what debits and credits are and how they work in the general accounting process. In particular, many people believe a debit increases something and a credit decreases something. This is false. Simply put, you enter debits on the left-hand side of the balance sheet and credits on the right-hand side. Perhaps a bit more complicated to understand is that debits and credits often convey slightly different information when one is speaking about assets, liabilities, owner's equity, revenue, or expenses. Not to worry; in this chapter, we will look at some examples of debiting and crediting an account to clarify the meaning of these terms.

Example 1

A nursing facility purchases five new beds at a total cost of $3,000. The new beds are a supply for the facility and therefore are also a tangible element that the facility now owns—in other words, they are an asset. When you debit an asset, it increases the asset accounts, and when you credit an asset account, it decreases this account. As such, for this transaction, our account and accounting transaction would look like this:

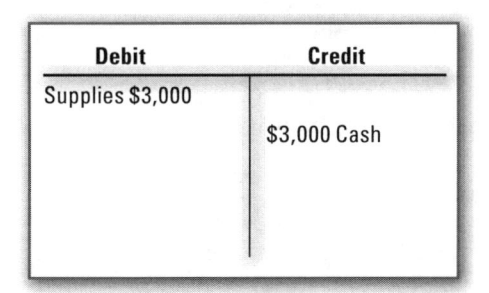

Debit	Credit
Supplies $3,000	
	$3,000 Cash

Notice in the preceding figure that the facility gained an asset: the supplies (beds). Because of this, we enter the supplies as a debit balance, on the left-hand side of the T-account. However, the facility paid cash for the supplies, and consistent with the rules of double-entry accounting, we simultaneously enter the $3,000 cash the facility paid for the supplies as a credit balance, on the right-hand side of the balance sheet.

CHAPTER 3

Now, what if the facility sold its beds to another facility for $3,000? Such an entry would look like this:

Debit	Credit
$3,000 Cash	
	Supplies $3,000

In this case, the supplies have been credited, because the beds the facility initially acquired as an asset gained are no longer part of the facility. However, look at what happened with the cash. Cash is also an asset. In the first T-account, cash was a credit entry because it was reduced. However, on the second T-account above, cash was a debit entry because it was increased. Since the facility sold the beds, the facility obtained cash from sales of the beds and therefore cash was debited. Remember, we are using these examples based on the accrual method of accounting. Consequently, even if the cash was not paid at the time the beds were sold, the transaction would still be posted on the account simultaneously with the sale of the beds, and even if the cash for the sale of the beds was not received until the following month, the cash was realized when the beds were sold and would be posted to the account when they were sold and not when the cash was received.

Example 2

A local hospital purchases new 3-D echocardiogram equipment at a cost of $200,000. The hospital purchased the equipment on account, and therefore it becomes an account payable. An account payable is a liability because it is money owed, and thus it is a debt for the facility in which the creditors have a claim on the equity of the facility. This means they have a stake in the facility to obtain their money if legal action or bankruptcy happens. Liabilities usually have a credit balance; a debit decreases liability and a credit increases liability. Therefore, this transaction would appear on the balance sheet as follows:

Debit	Credit
$200,000 Equipment	
	$200,000 Accounts Payable

THE FINANCIAL CAPTAIN: THE BALANCE SHEET

The preceding figure demonstrates that the hospital acquired capital: the 3-D echocardiogram equipment. This equipment is also an asset, and consistent with an asset added to the facility, it was recorded as a debit entry. However, the hospital purchased the equipment on account for $200,000, thus creating an outstanding account that the hospital must pay to the equipment supplier, which is a liability. An account payable is a liability, because the facility now owes creditors that have a legal claim against the facility's equity.

Now let's say the hospital pays the equipment supplier in full for the equipment it purchased. The entry for this transaction would look like the following:

Debit	Credit
$200,000	
Accounts Payable	
	$200,000
	Cash

Let's examine what transpired. Remember, crediting a liability increases the liability, whereas debiting a liability decreases the liability. The account payable was paid off, which in turn decreased the liability; hence, we have a debit entry. But again, cash was credited. Cash is an asset, and because it was disbursed to pay for the account receivable, it was reduced, and therefore it becomes a credit entry, reducing this asset.

Example 3

A sub-acute care facility enhances its physical therapy room at an expense of $100,000. An expense is entered on the debit side of the T-account, demonstrating the accounting transaction. Debiting an expense increases the expense, whereas crediting an expense decreases the expense. Here's how the entry for this transaction would look:

Debit	Credit
$100,000	
Physical Therapy Expense	
	$100,000
	Accounts Payable

Finance, Budgeting & Quantitative Analysis: A Primer for Nursing Home Administrators

CHAPTER 3

The expense is a debit balance. It is an expense the facility has accrued, and thus it is added to the expenses that already exist.

Now let's say that the $100,000 expense was paid on the account. An account payable, as noted earlier, is a liability. In this case, expenses as well as liabilities have increased. Again, the crediting of liabilities reflects the increase in liabilities. However, now the expense is paid and the following entry transpires:

Debit	Credit
$100,000 Accounts Payable	
	$100,000 Cash

Example 4

A skilled nursing facility receives a Medicare check for $90,000 for services rendered for three residents. Since the services were already rendered and the facility's accounts were already credited, the Medicare funds are cash that must be entered into each of the three resident's accounts and posted appropriately with a reversal entry. For simplicity, only one account is shown in this example, but it would actually require a posting to three separate accounts—documenting reimbursement for the services rendered to each of the three residents. For this example, each resident received $30,000 of the total $90,000.

Debit	Credit
$30,000 Cash for resident X	
	$30,000 Accounts Receivable for resident X

In the previously described entry, when the services were rendered for resident X, the facility would have debited the resident's accounts receivable and credited cash. Now, the Medicare check has been sent to the facility for the services rendered, $30,000 for each of the three residents, for a total of $90,000. What exists above for one resident is basically a reversal of the original accounting transaction.

THE FINANCIAL CAPTAIN: THE BALANCE SHEET

Example 5

A long-term care facility sends out its bills for the month of March on April 1. When the bookkeeper entered that transaction into the account of one of the facility's patients, Mrs. Doe, the entry was for the amount of receivables due for the month of March, the period of time that the $3,000 for services rendered was realized.

Debit	Credit
$3,000 Accounts Receivable	
	$3,000 Cash

Although the bookkeeper made this notation into the patient's account in March, this is still considered revenue or money coming in but not actually received yet. However, consistent with the GAAP and the accrual accounting method, the revenue was realized in March and that is when it is entered. This transaction also demonstrates two assets: debiting accounts receivable and increasing this asset, and crediting cash and decreasing this asset. For example, our accounts receivable account described above was increased by $3,000. Conversely, if our cash account had $40,000 in it, the $3,000 paid out would receive that account down to $37,000.

A week later, on April 8, John Doe came into the facility to pay his mother's bill for March. At this point, the bookkeeper simply makes a reversal entry. The revenue is still unchanged, but the two asset accounts demonstrate a reversed entry.

Debit	Credit
$3,000 Cash	
	$3,000 Accounts Receivable

Finance, Budgeting & Quantitative Analysis: A Primer for Nursing Home Administrators

CHAPTER 3

Accounting for Accruals and Deferrals

Transactions that are not always accounted for or not fully realized often exist. Nevertheless, these transactions have to be recorded in some form. Healthcare administrators commonly reconcile their organization's monthly finances, and to do so, administrators must account for any accruals and deferrals.

A deferral records an expense or revenue in a manner that delays the recognition of the expense or revenue. In other words, the recognition of an expense or revenue is delayed and a transaction is made to reflect this delayed realization. There are two types of deferrals: deferred expenses and deferred revenues. Deferred expenses are initially recorded as assets, but over time they are realized as expenses. A common deferred expense is prepaid insurance. This form of insurance is initially recorded as an asset that is amortized over a period of time. A prepaid insurance premium of $1,200 per year is initially recorded as an asset, but over the following 12-month period, $100 is expensed each month for a total of $1,200.

Deferred revenues are initially recorded as liabilities but are realized as revenues over time. The full revenue amount is paid at one time, but the revenue has not been earned at the time of payment. The fee for an attorney's annual retainer that organizations often pay is an example of this type of deferral.

Accruals are adjustments that healthcare administrators most commonly address, especially as part of month-end closing reports. There are two types of accruals: accrued expenses and accrued revenues. Accrued expenses are expenses that have been incurred but have not been recorded. A common accrued expense is employee wages. Although they are accrued, employee wages are not typically paid out fully at the end of each month. Nevertheless, these wages are accrued expenses, or liabilities to the company, that must be accounted for to accurately reflect the end-of-month reconciliation. For example, consider a pay period that ranges from March 25 to April 8. In this case, the month-end closing report for March must reflect six days of accrued wage expense that has not been paid out by the end of that month.

Accrued revenues are assets that have been earned but not recorded as an accounting transaction. For example, consider a facility that has provided healthcare services to a resident in a given month, but the resident's insurance company was not billed at the time services were provided. The revenue was accrued at the time of service, but cash for the resident was not received until after the insurance company was billed. Another example is a facility that rents out part of the building to another company that provides renal/dialysis services. The renting of the space is often an accrued form of revenue in which the facility realized the rent revenue by providing the space but is not paid until the end of each month.

4 The Accounting Cycle

The accounting cycle usually begins with a transaction. A transaction is any type of accounting activity that has transpired. The term transaction connotes that the activity is typically bilateral and not unilateral. For example, a healthcare facility buys medical supplies from a medical supply company. The transaction is between the healthcare facility and the supply company.

After the transaction takes place, it is documented. The documentation is usually made in a journal of some kind. For example, it could be made in the facility's general journal, a cash receipts journal, or a cash disbursement journal. Facilities use other types of journals in addition to these; regardless of the type, it is important that the transaction is entered into the correct journal (Allen 1997). This process of entering information into a journal is called journalizing. Remember, the accounting process works on both sides of the transaction. Not only are you documenting and journalizing your transaction, but the other party is documenting its transaction with you as well. Transactions are usually journalized on the basis of the accrual accounting method and the double-entry, debit, and credit system.

Most journals have an area that deals with postings, in which you enter the account number indicating the ledger account in which you will also enter the transaction. Healthcare organizations usually have something called a chart of accounts that lists all of their asset, liability, expense, revenue, and capital accounts. These accounts are usually numbered. For example, say the first 10 accounts are asset accounts. Accounts 11–18 may be liability accounts. Accounts 19–25 may be revenue accounts, 26–35 expense accounts, and 36–40 capital accounts. After journalizing the transaction, you post the transaction to its respective ledger account. The following example shows a simple journal format with posting information:

Date	Account Name	Post	Debit	Credit
3/20/2012	Supplies	5	$100	
	Cash	1		$100

CHAPTER 4

In the preceding example, the information has been journalized, and as you can see it affects the Supplies account and the Cash account. Within the ledger, the accounts are represented by their posting numbers. Therefore, the transaction now is posted to the Supplies account and the Cash account. The following is the entry:

	Supply Account				Cash Account	
	Debit	Credit			Debit	Credit
3/20/2012	$100			3/20/2012		$100

Now let's say that on March 25, the company bought additional medical supplies on credit for $2,000. The following entries were journalized and then posted to the Supplies account and accounts payable:

Date	Account Name	Post	Debit	Credit
3/25/2012	Supplies	5	$2,000	
	Accts. Payable	12		$2,000

	Supply Account				Accounts Payable	
	Debit	Credit			Debit	Credit
3/20/2012	$100			3/25/2012		$2000
3/25/2012	$2000					

Now let's assume the facility paid off its accounts payable on March 31. The facility would make the following entries. First, it would journalize the entries and then post them to their respective posted accounts.

Date	Account Name	Post	Debit	Credit
3/31/2012	Accts. Payable	12	$2,000	
	Cash	1		$2,000

	Accounts Payable				Cash Account	
	Debit	Credit			Debit	Credit
3/25/2012		$2000		3/25/2012		$100
3/31/2012	$2000			3/31/2012		$2,000

THE ACCOUNTING CYCLE

Closing Accounts

All the accounts we have discussed thus far eventually have to be closed. Revenue and expense accounts are closed at the end of the accounting cycle, which is usually the end of the month, through the use of the revenue and expense summary. All revenue and expense accounts are reduced to zero at the end of the accounting period. After each revenue and expense account is closed, it is transferred to the revenue and expense summary, after which the revenue and expense summary is closed to the retained earnings account. This sounds somewhat complicated, and for the most part it is, especially when dealing with a large number of accounts. But the concept can be simplified by demonstrating it through the use of a few accounts. The accounting itself is not difficult, but it is procedural.

Individual revenue and expense accounts

The first step is to close the individual revenue and expense accounts. Because revenue accounts normally have credit balances, we will have to make a debit entry on the opposite side for an amount that equals the right side. Conversely, when closing out expense accounts that normally have debit balances, we have to make a credit entry that equals the left side and that balances the account to zero. In the following example, we will use two revenue and two expense accounts to demonstrate this process. Also, we will demonstrate the closing entry to close the account to zero through the use of boldface numbers. It should be mentioned that Medicare revenue will usually be placed in the individual resident's account instead of having an entire account for Medicare, but for simplicity, Medicare is used in the following example.

	Medicare Revenue				Medicaid Revenue	
	Debit	Credit			Debit	Credit
3/06/2012		$80,000	3/08/2012			$150,000
3/31/2012	**$80,000**		3/25/2012			$170,000
			3/31/2012		**$320,000**	

	Wages Expense				Medical Supplies Expense	
	Debit	Credit			Debit	Credit
3/08/2012	$90,000		3/05/2012		$10,000	
3/22/2012	$88,000		3/20/2012		$25,000	
3/31/2012		**$178,000**	3/25/2012		$20,000	
			3/31/2012			**$55,000**

Finance, Budgeting & Quantitative Analysis: A Primer for Nursing Home Administrators

CHAPTER 4

As you can see by the bolded entries, we close the revenue accounts in the left-sided entry to leave the balance at zero, and we balance out the expense accounts by entering a right-sided entry, leaving the accounts balanced to zero. Because the accounts have now been closed, the next step is to enter the individual accounts into a revenue and expense summary. For revenue accounts, the revenue is now debited to the revenue and expense summary, whereas expenses are credited on the revenue and expense summary. Again, using an example will help to demonstrate this procedure.

Revenue and Expense Summary (For Revenue)		Debit	Credit
3/31/2012	Medicare Revenue	$ 80,000	
	Revenue and Expense Summary		$ 80,000
3/31/2012	Medicaid Revenue	**$320,000**	
	Revenue and Expense Summary		$320,000
Revenue and Expense Summary (For Expenses)		**Debit**	**Credit**
3/31/2012	Revenue and Expense Summary	$178,000	
	Wage Expense		$178,000
3/31/2012	Revenue and Expense Summary	$ 55,000	
	Medical Supplies Expense		$ 55,000

The final step is to subtract the expenses from the revenue and post the sum to the capital or retained earnings account. If the balance from the revenue and expense summary is a revenue-based balance, where revenue exceeds expenses, the entry is to debit the revenue and expense summary and credit the revenue balance. If you have an expense-based balance, where expenses exceed revenue, you debit the retained earnings and credit the revenue and expense summary. The following example shows how this process works:

Total Revenue = $400,000 – Total Expenses = $233,000 = $167,000			
Retained Earnings		Debit	Credit
3/31/2012	Revenue and Expense Summary	$167,000	
	Retained Earnings		$167,000

The preceding example demonstrates an entry in which there was a net profit and revenue exceeded expenses. However, if expenses exceeded revenue using the same numbers, the entry would be reversed.

THE ACCOUNTING CYCLE

			Debit	Credit
3/31/2012	Retained Earnings		$167,000	
	Revenue and Expense Summary			$167,000

| Revenue and Expense Summary || | Retained Earnings ||
Debit	Credit		Debit	Credit
3/31/2012 $233,000	$400,000	3/01/2012		$250,000
		3/31/2012		$167,000
				$417,000

The preceding example demonstrates the postings into the revenue and expense summary and, subsequently, the final posting to the retained earnings summary. Because revenue exceeded expenses, the $167,000 of net profit is posted to the retained earnings as a credit balance. The $250,000 was retained earnings that are already in the account. At the bottom there is a balance of $417,000 of retained earnings. However, if we use the same numbers but now have revenue of $233,000 and expenses of $400,000, we would have a net loss of ($167,000). If this had happened, the revenue and expense summary would show a debit of $400,000 and a credit of $233,000. We would have posted this loss to the retained earnings statement as a debit entry of $167,000 to retained earnings, which in turn would have created a balance of $83,000.

Writing Off Uncollectible Accounts

Writing off an uncollectible debt, especially in long-term healthcare, is not a preferred means for closing an account. Especially during this period when Medicaid and Medicare cutbacks have ensued, collecting on your accounts receivable is imperative. Yet, writing off accounts that cannot be collected does happen.

To avoid having to write off an account, you should maintain frequent contact with your *accounts aging document*. This is an important document that you can produce with your accounting software. Watch for those accounts that go past 30 days. The longer an account is delinquent, the more difficult it is to collect, especially in totality, on the account.

If you cannot avoid having to write off an account, the following information should help you with this process.

CHAPTER 4

Reminder notices

Look at the accounts aging document a couple times per month to help consolidate into memory those accounts that are delinquent and need to be addressed quickly. Do not be afraid to send reminder notices to individuals about unpaid accounts, but be courteous and respectful. People do forget, and usually those that are not delinquency risks will address the issue after the first reminder letter and often will do so apologetically.

Collection agencies and legal action

If the aging continues without any payment to the account, your next notification should be more firm, stating that payment is needed, with a reminder of the amount that is due. Continue to be tactful and considerate, but remain firm and address the next course of action that will be taken if the account remains unpaid.

If nothing happens, it is time to initiate the course of action that you previously described. You may have to contact a collection agency or take some other form of legal action. For example, you may have a resident whose family member is not paying the resident's patient pay amount, which is the amount the resident is responsible for even if Medicaid is paying for the patient's long-term care. Possibly a family member who is the responsible party or guardian now is responsible for paying this because the resident can no longer do so due to his or her level of infirmity. If this person is not paying, or if he or she is misappropriating the resident's funds that were stipulated to be paid to your facility, your facility may have to petition the probate court or have your corporate legal counsel address this issue, which could lead to the court appointing another personal guardian and/or conservator to help address payment of the facility in a timely manner.

You can take other types of legal action to help your facility acquire the delinquent funds. However, again, it is important that the bookkeeper in the facility and the administrator pay close attention at regular intervals to aging accounts and act on those accounts promptly and in a consistent manner so that legal action is used only as a final recourse.

Writing off an account

If you have exhausted all avenues and you cannot collect on a patient account through any apparent means, you must write off the account. Writing off a patient account usually has greater financial implications for a nursing facility than for a large Fortune 500 company.

THE ACCOUNTING CYCLE

For example, writing off a patient account of $20,000 means you have $20,000 less to spend for the other residents at your facility. Therefore, you should do this only as a last resort, after you have tried all other measures to collect the receivables that are due to the facility. When you do need to write off an uncollectible account, you can do so in a few different ways. However, this book demonstrates only one, because write-offs are usually the purview of the accountant and not the administrator. Yet the administrator often has strong input into this decision and should understand some of the basic accounting procedures for writing off an account.

With that said, a facility can directly write off an account by using the following entries:

Example of a Direct Write-Off

Ms. Jane Doe had uncollected receivables totaling $20,000. The nursing facility was not able to collect this debt and ended up writing off Ms. Doe's account.

General Journal

		Debit	Credit
4/20/2012	Uncollectible Acct. Expense	$20,000	
	Accts. Receivable, Jane Doe		$20,000

Working Capital

An important analytical financial concept that an administrator needs to understand is working capital, which is defined as current assets minus current liabilities.

Working Capital = Current Assets – Current Liabilities

Working capital is not a ratio, but it is important because it deals with the business' liquidity, or the assets and liabilities that are liquid or can be converted to cash quickly. These assets and liabilities are part of the daily healthcare environment, and they account for many of the obligations that must be addressed or worked with by relying on liquid assets—thus the concept of working capital. You may be making a profit as a company, but there could be a considerable amount of wealth held within long-term assets, which fail to have the liquidity of current assets and subsequently fail to have quick conversion to cash (working capital). This can cause a significant problem in paying your bills, especially many of your short-term obligations that you have to creditors.

CHAPTER 4

In reality, you want to have enough current assets to meet your current liabilities. If your current liabilities extend beyond your current assets, you do not have enough liquidity to meet your short-term obligations. That can be a major problem. Often, if this is not corrected, your continued inability to meet your current obligations compounds the facility's debt. This can be the start of runaway debt problems that can be difficult to get under control. Current liabilities that dramatically exceed the level of current assets can raise major questions regarding your organization's solvency.

Conversely, what if you had $2 million of current assets and $1 million of current liabilities? Does this make you feel better? It should, given that your current assets exceed your current liabilities by $1 million. You are in a better position than if you were overcome by debt and had short-term obligations that you could not meet. Yet, you may have too much working capital sitting idle. Possibly, you could divert some of this working capital to pay some long-term debt, and you could invest in money market securities or other capital that may enhance the organization's financial growth. Therefore, just as not having enough liquidity can be a problem, having too much of a good thing sitting idle can also be problematic.

Net Operating Margin

A facility's net operating margin can add a sizable amount of information regarding the facility's solvency. The net operating margin is defined as the net operating revenue minus net operating expenses divided by net operating revenue (Allen, 1997).

$$\text{Net Operating Margin} = \frac{\text{Net Operating Revenue} - \text{Net Operating Expenses}}{\text{Net Operating Revenue}}$$

To better understand the concept of net operating margin, it helps to remember the difference between operating and nonoperating revenue and expenses discussed earlier. In the income statement used previously, the operating revenue was $340,000 and the operating expenses were $283,000. Plugging these numbers into the preceding equation demonstrates the following:

$$\text{Net Operating Margin} = \frac{\$340{,}000 - \$283{,}000}{\$340{,}000} = +16.76\%$$

THE ACCOUNTING CYCLE

In the previously described example, remember to multiply the sum of the numerator divided by the dominator by 100 to convert the number to a percentage. This example shows a pretty strong operating margin. Most healthcare facilities would feel satisfied if that was their regular operating margin. However, many actually have negative operating margins, which, given the industry, is not all that rare. Therefore, it is very important to document whether it is a positive or negative operating margin by placing a positive or negative sign in front of the percentage.

Current Ratio and Debt-to-Equity Ratio

Two other important ratios, often referred to as liquidity ratios because they look at the potential for quick conversion of cash and cash-like resources to meet outstanding obligations, are the *current ratio* and the *debt-to-equity ratio*.

You can determine the current ratio as follows:

$$\text{Current Ratio} = \frac{\text{Current Assets}}{\text{Current Liabilities}}$$

This ratio demonstrates your current assets compared to your current liabilities. Anything less than 1 should raise questions regarding the facility's solvency and its ability to meet its short-term obligations in a timely manner. When a facility is setting up accounts on credit, a current ratio of less than 1 could be problematic, especially if there is a history of poor liquidity (Silbiger 1993). A facility with a ratio greater than 1 has a level of liquidity that will enable it to meet its short-term obligations.

You can determine the debt-to-equity ratio, sometimes called the debt-to-net worth ratio, as follows:

$$\text{Debt to Equity} = \frac{\text{Total Debt}}{\text{Owner's or Shareholder's Equity}}$$

A lower debt-to-equity ratio helps to illuminate the company's liquidity and hence its ability to meet its obligations. When the debt-to-equity ratio is high, the facility becomes a risk company, and setting up new accounts on credit will be difficult. Furthermore, the existing risk lays a heavy burden on the facility's creditors. Conversely, a lower debt-to-equity ratio demonstrates that the facility is in a less precarious position, especially in terms of meeting its obligations. Using the balance sheet from Chapter 2 as an example, the facility's total debt-to-equity ratio would be 23.77, indicating that a fairly high risk may exist for creditors. Such numbers probably will not inspire confidence for banks if the facility tries to obtain a loan.

Capitalization Ratio

You must be careful when using only one ratio to make broad generalizations about your facility's financial health. For example, when trying to convey the financial solvency of your facility, one particular ratio may raise eyebrows. But to get a complete picture of where your facility stands, the administrator and other financial personnel must examine many dimensions of the facility's financial position. Therefore, numerous and diverse types of financial ratios must be examined to garner a more precise understanding of the facility's financial position.

Silbiger (1993) speaks about two important ratios that many healthcare administrators should consider. *Capitalization ratios* help you to examine how your facility is funding itself and how burdened it is with debt, which in turn can interfere with appropriate funding. One important capitalization ratio is *financial leverage*, which indicates the level of debt the facility is assuming compared to its owner's investments. The financial leverage ratio is as follows:

$$\text{Financial Leverage} = \frac{\text{Total Liabilities} + \text{Owner's Equity}}{\text{Owner's Equity}}$$

Given the balance sheet that we used earlier for XYZ Nursing Home in Chapter 2, the financial leverage would equal 24.77, a ratio that is high and that demonstrates that the facility is heavily leveraged. Silbiger (1993) states that a ratio greater than 2 demonstrates an extensive use of debt; this means the facility is highly leveraged against the owner's financial investments being made to maintain adequate solvency. In other words, you have too much debt working against you. Total liabilities have to be reduced to help you in the long run.

Another capitalization ratio is the *long-term debt-to-capital ratio*. You can determine this ratio via the following equation:

$$\text{Long-Term Debt to Capital} = \frac{\text{Long-Term Debt}}{\text{Liabilities} + \text{Owner's Equity}}$$

THE ACCOUNTING CYCLE

Again, using the XYZ Nursing Home balance sheet from earlier, we see that the long-term debt equals $5 million and the total liabilities and owner's equity equal $7.06 million. When we plug these numbers into the equation, the result is 0.708, which again is a high number, indicating that long-term debt comprises slightly more than 70% of the facility's total liability and owner's equity. Silbiger (1993) states that a ratio of 50% or greater indicates a high level of debt. Our fictional financial indicators up to this point have not presented an inspiring representation of this facility and its financial status.

Average Collection Period Ratio and Accounts Payable Average Payment Period Ratio

At this point, we should examine some important activity or efficiency ratios. These ratios help to demonstrate how well a facility is conducting its daily activities, especially in terms of collecting money that is owed to it in a timely manner, as well as paying money to its creditors in a timely manner. Two important ratios in this category are the *average collection period ratio* and the *accounts payable average payment period ratio*. You can calculate these ratios in a few different ways, and merchandising companies often will use slightly different equations to calculate them. This book will rely on Allen (1997) and his equations for figuring out these two important efficiency ratios for healthcare facilities.

The first ratio, the average collection period ratio, examines how efficient your company is at collecting the payments that are due for services rendered. The following is the equation:

$$\text{Average Collection Period Ratio} = \frac{365 \times \text{Accounts Receivables}}{\text{Net Operating Revenue}}$$

Let's say that after you multiplied your accounts receivable by 365 days and then divided that by your net operating revenue, you came up with a number of 62.3. This means your collection period, on average, is slightly more than two months. With such a high average, you run the risk of compiling debt that you cannot pay, because although you may have realized the asset, the facility may not have received the payment.

Therefore, your short-term obligations will suffer if you do not have the resources that are owed to you for available deployment. You should try to keep your average close to 30 days and limit any increasing

CHAPTER 4

deviations from that benchmark 30-day period. This is why it is so important to maintain a close and frequent inspection of the accounts aging document.

A second important efficiency indicator is the accounts payable average payment period ratio. Just as your facility expects efficient and prompt remittance of accounts receivable, your creditors also expect prompt, timely remittance of payment that is due to them. The following is how to figure out the accounts payable average payment period ratio:

$$\text{Accounts Payable Average Payment Period Ratio} = \frac{365 \times \text{Accounts Payable}}{\text{Supplies Expense}}$$

Most accounts come with terms, which are usually 30 days from the day of receipt. Waiting too long to pay your suppliers can cause a number of problems:

1. It places you on poor terms with your creditors, who may cancel your contracts or remove you from their credit terms and place you on cash-on-delivery status

2. Your credit standing is influenced dramatically and can affect your business when you try to open and enter into future contracts

3. You may compound your debt, not only on each account for its respective supplier but also as an aggregate

As we already examined with capitalization ratios, adding too much debt may inadequately leverage your facility to such a high level that you reach a cycle where you fail to meet your short-term as well as long-term obligations.

Try to keep your payables average to 30–45 days. This inspires confidence in your current creditors as well as any future ones, and it prevents you from getting into the "catch-up" cycle, in which you're always trying to catch up with payments. If this starts to happen and you have entered this catch-up cycle, you probably will continue to be plagued with trying to catch up on your payments. Furthermore, when entering into a new contract, do not be afraid to negotiate terms. Especially if you feel that certain terms are too stringent, try to negotiate terms that are more compatible with the solvency of your facility.

THE ACCOUNTING CYCLE

Return on Assets and Return on Equity

Owners of a facility often want to know about the facility's profitability, and the administrator or accountant may have to provide them with information regarding their return on assets (ROA) or return on equity (ROE). The following demonstrates how both of these profitability ratios are determined:

$$ROA = \frac{Net\ Income}{Total\ Assets} \qquad ROE = \frac{Net\ Income}{Owner's\ Equity}$$

Given our examples of using the income statement and balance sheet for our fictional company, XYZ Nursing Home, from Chapter 2, the ROA = +0.28 and the ROE = +7.02. Often, ROE is viewed more seriously as a benchmark for a successful company. Are these ratios demonstrating a good or bad financial disposition for this company? It is difficult to say just by examining the ratios. One has to be aware of the industry averages in this area, especially as they relate to profitability. In other words, depending on your industry, these may be terrible or they may be consistent with industry profitability standards.

Given the healthcare industry in general, as well as long-term care in particular, profitability has not been great, and often modest returns on assets and equity that would make others in sales, communications, and merchandising shudder may be viewed as successful.

Other Useful Ratios

In the austere reimbursement environment of the healthcare industry, many administrators, especially in long-term care, are paying close attention to their census and how it relates to the spread of cost over a period of time. Many administrators often speak about the PPD cost, or their cost per patient day.

A useful measure is to examine the census occupancy over a one-month period as it relates to the expenses that have been realized for that month. For example, let's say that during April, a 90-bed facility averaged 82.57 residents. This is an average occupancy rate for the month of 91.74%. Also, during that month, the facility had $275,000 in expenses. To calculate the average cost per patient or resident day, we would use the following formula:

Monthly Expenses / Number of Days in the Month / Occupancy Rate for the Month

Finance, Budgeting & Quantitative Analysis: A Primer for Nursing Home Administrators

CHAPTER 4

This states that monthly expenses are divided by the number of days in the month. This answer is then divided by the occupancy rate. Because the monthly expenses were $275,000, we divide this by the 30-day month of April. This leaves 9166.67, which in turn is divided by the occupancy rate for the month, 91.74. The average cost per patient (resident) day, therefore, is $99.92.

At times a facility makes a capital expenditure, and such an investment often is followed by a question: "How long will it take for the facility to get back what it is putting out?" We cannot answer this question in a simple, straightforward way. Yet, for investments that are not extensive, in which cost is not required to be estimated over a large number of years, we can calculate the payback period. To do this, we divide the total investment by the annual savings to determine the number of years in which the investment will be fully achieved:

$$\text{Payback Period} = \frac{\text{Total Investment}}{\text{Annual Savings}}$$

For example, say a long-term care facility invests in equipment costing $10,000 with an annual savings of $7,000. This equals a payback period of 1.4285, which means the facility will get its investment back in less than roughly 18 months. I use the term *roughly* because the payback period does not take into consideration the time value of money and how it changes from one year to another. So, as a rule of thumb, the payback period works better for short-term investments than for long-term investments. This is because it holds the value of money constant without adjusting it for the varying time periods.

Depreciation and Depreciation Expense

Depreciation spreads the useful cost of an asset over a number of years, often determined by the IRS for tax purposes. Most of the long-term assets a company owns, with the exception of land, experience wear and tear and become outdated, which consequently reduces the useful life of this type of asset.

Depreciation is also a noncash expense. Although a monetary reduction in the asset's book value (the asset's worth after determining its depreciation) demonstrates a monetary reduction in its current value, the expense is created through the wear and tear of using the asset, its obsolescence with time, and similar factors, which are not cash-based expenses but nonetheless are expenses that must be placed in monetary terms. Remember that Generally Accepted Accounting Principles (GAAP) adhere to accounting being done objectively, and depreciation helps to quantify a noncash expense.

THE ACCOUNTING CYCLE

The straight-line method

Probably the most common procedure for determining depreciation is the straight-line method. This method is fairly straightforward. It takes the original price that was paid for the asset, minus any *salvage value* (residual value left when all depreciation is complete), and divides the original price by the number of expected years of usefulness. Remember, each asset is usually not depreciated randomly, regardless of the method of depreciation used, but usually a set number of years for usefulness is established for particular assets.

As an example, let's say that XYZ Nursing Home buys a van to take residents out for trips and activities. The cost of the van is $22,000. The van's salvage value is $2,000 and it has a useful life of five years. The following is how you would determine the van's depreciation value using the straight-line method of depreciation:

> Cost = $22,000 – $2,000 = $20,000 / 5 years = $4,000 for each of the next 5 years

This means that for each of the next five years, the depreciation expense will be $4,000 annually. For accounting purposes, you would set up an account for the van, possibly under the facility's Equipment account, a depreciation expense, and a contra-asset account called accumulated depreciation. But for this example, let's look at the years and the accumulated depreciation and book value.

Year	Amount Depreciated	Accumulated Depreciation	Book Value
1	$4,000	$ 4,000	$18,000
2	$4,000	$ 8,000	$14,000
3	$4,000	$12,000	$10,000
4	$4,000	$16,000	$ 6,000
5	$4,000	$20,000	$ 2,000

The accelerated depreciation method

Contrary to the straight-line method that spreads cost equally over a number of years, *the accelerated depreciation method* depreciates greater amounts of the asset during early years and lesser amounts during later years. There are a couple of different approaches that can be used in calculating the accelerated form of depreciation. We will address two of them in this section: the sum-of-years method and the double-declining balance method.

CHAPTER 4

The *sum-of-years method of depreciation* starts by summing the total number of years of the asset's useful life. For example, the life of the van mentioned in the preceding section was five years, so the sum of the years would be 1 + 2 + 3 + 4 + 5 = 15. The sum, 15, would be the denominator, and each year would be the numerator. When the respective year is divided by the sum, it provides a percentage of the total cost that will be depreciated for the year. The following demonstrates this process using the same $22,000 van purchase:

Year	Rate	Annual Dep.	Acc Dep.	Book Value
1	5/15 = 0.3333	$7,332.60	$ 7,332.60	$14,667.40
2	4/15 = 0.26666	$5,866.52	$13,199.12	$ 8,800.88
3	3/15 = 0.20	$4,400	$17,599.12	$ 4,400.88
4	2/15 = 0.13333	$2,933.26	$20,532.38	$ 1,467.62
5	1/15 = 0.06666	$1,466.52	$21,998.90	$ 1.10

Notice the difference in the depreciation schedule. Almost 80% of the depreciation occurred within the first three years. This is different from the equal amount that was spread over the five years with the straight-line method.

The *double-declining balance method* uses the straight-line method of depreciation, doubling that percentage and applying the percentage to the new book value to get the depreciation for the year. Using our example of the $22,000 purchase of a van with a salvage value of $2,000, the straight-line method depreciated the asset by the same dollar amount each year. In the example below, notice that when $4,400 is divided by $22,000 for a five-year period, the result is 20%. The following shows some simple math:

1. Straight-line depreciation is $4,400 per year, or 20% of the $22,000 without use of a salvage value

2. 20% × 2 = 40%

The following applies this depreciation process to the preceding example:

Year	Rate	Annual Dep	Acc Dep	Book Value
1	40%	$8,800	$ 8,800	$13,200
2	40%	$5,280	$14,080	$ 7,920
3	40%	$3,168	$17,248	$ 4,752
4	40%	$1,900.80	$19,148.80	$ 2,851.20
5	40%	$1,140.48	$20,289.28	$ 1,710.72

THE ACCOUNTING CYCLE

In this example, it can be seen that 78.4% of the depreciation was accounted for within the first three years. What method of depreciation should this facility use? Note that usually the administrator will not make this decision, nor will the administrator calculate depreciation. This is generally the responsibility of the accountant. However, often the accountant will meet with the administrator to discuss what depreciation method he or she will employ based on what he or she thinks will be best for the facility. Furthermore, some sources, such as cost accounting for Medicare and Medicaid, determine which method should be used.

5 Inventory

The IRS requires businesses to place a value on their inventory. It is difficult for a business to place a value on its current inventory, especially if the inventory is large and the business bought it at various times and for different prices. Therefore, accountants have devised some common procedures for approximating the value of current inventory. Once a business uses a particular procedure to evaluate its inventory, it should not use a different procedure. Deciding what procedure to use is best left to the business' accountant. Based on your facility's history, the accountant will be able to advise the best method for you to determine inventory valuation.

Probably the easiest inventory valuation method to understand is the *average cost method*. Simply put, the average cost method averages a business' remaining inventory by dividing the total cost by the units that are still in inventory and applies the average to the remaining units to determine the valuation of the current inventory.

Let's say your facility received shipments of briefs from two different suppliers with different unit prices, three times throughout the month. Each shipment delivers 1,000 briefs, at a total cost of $150 per shipment from Distributor A and $162 per shipment from Distributor B. There were 250 briefs in each of the four boxes that were delivered, for a *unit cost* (the box of 250 briefs) of $37.50 for Distributor A's shipment and $40.50 for Distributor B's shipment. At the beginning of the month, five boxes were in inventory from the prior month. At the end of the month, seven boxes were in inventory. The following is the breakdown:

Starting Inventory for the Month	5 units × 37.50 = $187.50
Delivery 1	4 units × 40.50 = $162
Delivery 2	4 units × 37.50 = $150
Delivery 3	4 units × 40.50 = $162

17 Units @ Average Cost = $38.91
Ending Inventory for the Month = 7 Units × $38.91 = $272.37

CHAPTER 5

Two other common inventory methods are the last-in-first-out (LIFO) method and the first-in-first-out (FIFO) method. The *FIFO method* assumes that the inventory that was first acquired will also be the first that is purchased or consumed. Another way you can look at this is that FIFO also means *last-in-still-here*, meaning that the last inventory purchased should still be in inventory because it will be the last used. When you use this method to determine inventory valuation, it will reflect the most recent cost of the inventory, which in turn can be misleading by portraying an early inventory cost that may be lower than the cost of later inventory items. The following example demonstrates this process:

Business supplies were bought three times during the month to add to the existing inventory. When a month-end inventory count was taken, 30 units of business supplies existed. What was the value of the ending inventory using the FIFO method of inventory valuation?

Starting Inventory		50 Units	@ $1 Cost per Unit	=	$ 50
4/02/2012	Purchase	100 Units	@ $1.25 Cost per Unit	=	$125
4/10/2012	Purchase	25 Units	@ $1.10 Cost per Unit	=	$ 27.50
4/20/2012	Purchase	25 Units	@ $1.50 Cost per Unit	=	$ 37.50
		200 Units			$240

Ending Inventory with 30 Units Left Equals:

25 Units	@ $1.50	=	$37.50
5 Units	@ $1.10	=	$ 5.50
30 Units			$43

Valuation of 30 Units of Ending Inventory = $43

The *LIFO method* of inventory valuation is the reverse of FIFO, assuming that the last items purchased will be the first to be used. In other words, the ending inventory valuation will be based on *first-in-still-here* thinking. Given that you are determining the valuation of your ending inventory on the cost of items that may have increased since you purchased them, the LIFO method may underestimate the value of your ending inventory. Let's use the same example we used previously to demonstrate the LIFO method.

INVENTORY

> Business supplies were bought three times during the month to add to the existing inventory. When a month-end inventory count was taken, 30 units of business supplies existed. What was the value of the ending inventory using the LIFO method of inventory valuation?
>
> | Starting Inventory | | 50 Units | @ $1 Cost per Unit | = | $ 50 |
> |---|---|---|---|---|---|
> | 4/02/2012 | Purchase | 100 Units | @ $1.25 Cost per Unit | = | $125 |
> | 4/10/2012 | Purchase | 25 Units | @ $1.10 Cost per Unit | = | $ 27.50 |
> | 4/20/2012 | Purchase | 25 Units | @ $1.50 Cost per Unit | = | $ 37.50 |
> | | | 200 Units | | | $240 |
>
> Inventory Used:
>
> | 25 Units | @ $1.50 | = | $ 37.50 |
> |---|---|---|---|
> | 25 Units | @ $1.10 | = | $ 27.50 |
> | 100 Units | @ $1.25 | = | $125 |
> | 20 Units | @ $1 | = | $ 20 |
> | 170 Units | | | $210 |
>
> Existing Inventory Valuation
>
> 30 Units @ $1 = $30

In this example, the facility consumed 170 units or $210 of its business supply inventory. Its ending inventory valuation was equal to 30 units left at a value of $1 per unit, or $30 total inventory valuation at the end of the month.

Procedures for Handling Cash Funds

Two important cash funds that are found in long-term care facilities are the petty cash fund and resident trust fund. The facility has to make sure it uses strong internal controls for cash to protect itself from possible misappropriation or skimming of funds. Both of these funds should be reconciled monthly, and the facility should:

1. Establish a routine for dealing with either account, such as assigning one person to do cash disbursements and receipts as well as make all deposits

2. Make sure all receipts and disbursements are signed and countersigned by the two transacting agents

3. Make sure those who receive and disburse are separate from those who do the accounting and reconciliation

CHAPTER 5

Petty cash funds

Petty cash funds are set up to provide a facility with a small amount of cash that it can access immediately for daily needs. Petty cash accounts for the facility and resident petty cash that are part of the resident trust are usually set up on an *imprest basis*. This means the funds are set up for a specific amount. For example, maybe your facility's petty cash fund is set at a monthly amount of $250 and its resident trust fund petty cash is set up at a monthly amount of $300.

Although larger businesses may place receipts and disbursement of these funds in their receipts or disbursements ledger, for a long-term care facility, it is probably best to have three separate journals, one for the facility petty cash and two others for the trust fund petty cash, to journalize in the first journal every disbursement and in the second journal any receipts made during the month.

The accounting entries in the journal would be made as follows:

Facility Petty Cash	Debit	Credit
Petty Cash	250	
Cash in Bank		250

Trust Fund Petty Cash	Debit	Credit
Trust Fund Petty Cash	300	
Cash in Bank		300

This is the initial entry to start up both accounts. You will not have to enter petty cash when replenishing the account, unless you decide to change the original amount to start the month. When replenishing the account you debit your disbursements, and when the account needs to be replenished, you credit cash in the bank.

Facility Petty Cash	Debit	Credit
Supplies	40	
Postage	10	
Computer Stand	80	
Posters	50	
Cash in Bank		180

Trust Fund Petty Cash	Debit	Credit
Ms. Jones	10	
Mr. Smith	20	
Ms. Smith	100	
Mr. Bob	50	
Ms. Doe	100	
Cash in Bank		280

INVENTORY

As mentioned earlier, the resident petty cash trust fund is slightly different from the facility petty cash fund. First, it is best to have two books for petty cash: one for the disbursements as shown earlier and another for any receipts, which family members often add to residents' trust fund accounts. This way, you have two daily journals of what is going in and what is going out regarding the two types of transactions.

Resident trust funds

However, once a person makes a resident trust fund transaction, after entering it into the resident trust disbursement or receipts journal, you should immediately enter it into the respective ledger that should be kept for each resident. Always make sure you enter the dates in the journals as well as in the ledgers so that you can better examine the documents if errors arise. Each resident should have a trust fund ledger that keeps a running tally of his or her trust fund accounts. The following is a quick summary of the resident trust fund transaction:

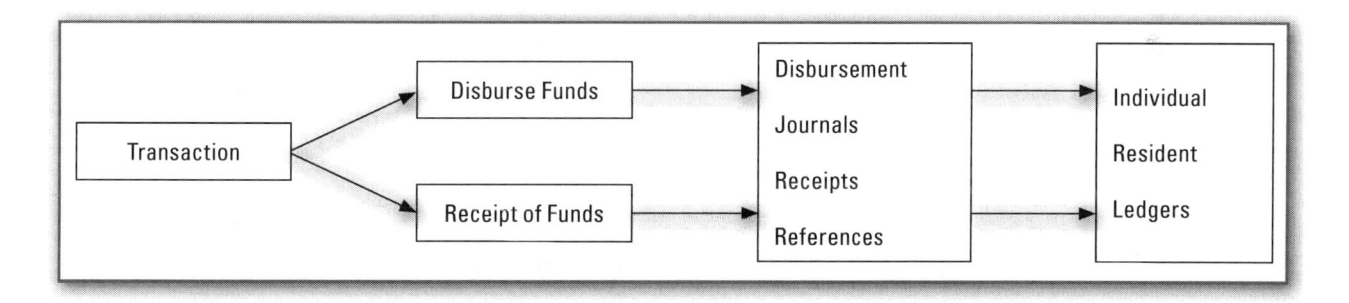

```
Transaction ──┬──► Disburse Funds    ──► Disbursement Journals  ──► Individual
              └──► Receipt of Funds  ──► Receipts References    ──► Resident Ledgers
```

The resident trust fund is an important internal accounting feature for the facility. All funds in excess of $50 ($100 for Medicare facilities only) must be deposited in an interest-bearing fund. The resident has the right to manage his or her financial affairs, and long-term care facilities cannot insist on residents depositing their funds with the facility, but when they do, the facility has to be able to provide adequate safeguards and management of funds. A nursing home's inadequate control of these funds is a violation of federal regulation F-Tag #158 and F-Tag #159.

The accounting procedure needs to be precise to make sure all trust money is accounted for, and this means that even when funds are placed in a pooled interest-bearing account, which most often they are, the interest should be factored in based on the pooled amount and the prevailing interest rate for that period. Federal regulations also state that quarterly statements should be provided to the resident or responsible parties, indicating the amount in the trust and any interest that has accrued. Many facilities will determine the interest on a quarterly basis. However, it is probably more efficient to do it monthly at the time the bank statement is received and to keep a running account of this in your computer spreadsheet.

CHAPTER 5

Also, by determining the interest monthly rather than quarterly, you can address any issues as well as possible errors on a more regular basis. Even though you do not have to provide the information to the resident or his or her family until the next quarter, doing your interest allocation monthly when you receive the bank statement keeps you current, makes allocation of interest easier, and makes your accounts current and more precise in dealing with these trust funds.

Surety Bonds and the Conveyance of Funds

Federal regulations state that within 30 days of a resident's death, that resident's funds, as well as an accounting of the resident's trust fund, should be conveyed to the resident's estate, the next of kin, or, if necessary, the probate jurisdiction. This is another good reason to address the trust monthly through the allocation of interest. It helps to make sure that the conveyance of funds upon death is being done in a timely manner. If not, regulators can cite the federal regulation F-Tag #160.

Also, administrators should always make sure that a surety bond exists in their facility and that it is adequate to cover the funds that are deposited in the trust. The surety bond is an assurance by the facility and insurance company that the facility can ensure coverage of trust funds on behalf of its residents if any loss of funds occurs. It is a necessary safeguard to protect residents' funds as well as to assist the facility if any unforeseen circumstances occur that could lead to the loss of such funds. Again, federal regulations mandate that an adequate surety bond be on file for resident fund protection.

Separation of duties

As mentioned earlier, important for internal control is the separation of those who handle receipt and disbursement of funds from those who handle accounting and reconciliation. Because the administrator is ultimately the chief financial officer of the long-term care facility, he or she should be responsible for making sure the accounting in this area is completed and done appropriately. A bookkeeper or office personnel could be assigned the duty of handling the facility trust or resident trust, but the administrator, through monthly accounting and reconciliation of these funds, should make sure that personnel who are handling disbursement and receipts of funds are journalizing and entering the appropriate funds in the correct manner. Again, addressing these funds, especially the resident trust fund, in an assiduous manner on a monthly basis helps to create an important oversight for the internal control of these funds.

INVENTORY

Banking and Reconciliation

A long-term care facility relies strongly on the bank or banks that it does business with, especially for deposits and check-writing privileges. First, healthcare facilities have to set up general accounts to deposit their cash assets. Furthermore, as previously mentioned, setting up trust accounts that are interest bearing for residents is important. In addition, facilities often have to have an in-house checking account, possibly for payments that need to be made or for transferring funds between accounts, to maintain proper management of these accounts.

It is imperative that bank account and checking account reconciliations are done promptly to:

1. Check for any mistakes the bank may have made

2. Check for any mistakes you may have made

3. Understand what the statements show and do not show

4. Reconcile the accounts so that you know your true cash balance

What sorts of things may reflect an inconsistency between your books and the bank statements you receive? As noted earlier, mistakes made by you or the bank could be the result of inconsistencies. Another issue may be deposits made that are in transit. This is a deposit made that for some reason was not recorded on the current monthly statement.

Outstanding checks or checks that were written but have not yet cleared the bank, and therefore are not found in the bank statement, will create a difference between the statement and your books. Overdrafts, which occur when checks are written for more than is in the account, as well as checks returned and labeled NSF (which stands for not sufficient funds), also create problems. Administrators need to spend less time on the formal accounting for these items and focus instead on how to deal with the reconciliation, which they have to address monthly to make sure the bank and the facility's books are correct. The following is a simple bank reconciliation statement:

CHAPTER 5

FIGURE 5.1
BANK RECONCILIATION FOR XYZ NURSING HOME

April 30, 2012

Balance per Bank	$5,000
Add: Deposit in Transit 4/30/12	$1,000
Subtotal	$6,000
Minus:	
Outstanding Checks:	
#250	$250
#260	$500
#270	$300
#280	$450
	$1,500
Adjusted Balance:	$4,500
Balance per Books	$3,500
Add: Unrecorded Automatic Deposit	$3,000
Collected Note with Interest	$1,000
Subtotal	$7,500
Minus:	
NSF (Jane Doe)	$2,500
Check #300 Transcription Error	$475
Collection Fee	$5
Service Charge	$20
	$3,000
Adjusted Balance:	$4,500

When doing the bank reconciliation, keep your checkbook in front of you as well as any deposit entries and receipts. Check off the checks the bank processed and highlight the check receipts that are not processed and are still outstanding. Develop a policy for outstanding checks. If the check has not been processed after 90 days, call the bank and cancel the check.

6 Planning and Budgeting

Planning is an essential function of all administrators, and it continues to play a major role in healthcare administration. Planning deals with delineating both the short-term and long-term paths that a business will follow and what procedures it will utilize to achieve its goal.

The Strategic Plan

The strategic plan is a plan that usually looks farther down the road, indicating what objectives the facility would like to achieve four, five, or even 10 years into the future. Typically, the strategic plan considers periods of five years for setting and obtaining strategic planning objectives (Tuller, 1997). Conversely, the tactical or business plan usually is based on a shorter period, generally one year, delineating specific objectives to be achieved within the upcoming fiscal year. Both types of planning are important in all types of business, and healthcare is no different. In this chapter, we will emphasize short-term planning, leading to the need to determine and construct an operating budget.

Tackling the Budget

A budget is a written plan that is formalized in an objective, quantifiable format. In other words, it lists your goals and states them in monetary terms (Mose, Jackson, & Downs, 1997). It provides an objective and concrete benchmark to determine how the business is operating over a specific period, usually the fiscal year for a healthcare facility. It therefore aids in creating an empirical monetary measurement of the health and well-being of your healthcare institution.

The budget you have created must be sound and well thought out for you to be able to determine your financial goals over the next fiscal year. Achieving or even exceeding your budgeted goals may hold little

CHAPTER 6

relevance if the budget was created in a cursory manner, leading to poorly objectified monetary goals that may be inconsistent with the facility's needs and with the industry and geographic region that harbors your facility.

Staffing and census budgets

Budgets are important for all phases of healthcare management. Budgets do not necessarily have to always address revenue, expenses, cash, and capital, all of which are budgetary features we will discuss in more detail shortly. Budgets can also address such things as hours of nursing care for each resident, or budgeted hours for dietary and housekeeping staffs, based on the census of the facility.

This is often necessary because the census is often a major driving force in determining cost. As much as 60%–70% of the cost to run a long-term care facility concerns labor costs. Although healthcare in itself is a service-intensive environment, long-term care facilities, especially skilled nursing facilities, have much more labor-intensive features that need to be addressed correctly and in accordance with the census.

If this is not done daily, it could lead to payroll expenses that exceed what is appropriately needed given the census in your facility. Because the Centers for Medicare & Medicaid Services (CMS) now mandates the posting of your daily census and the staff that your facility has for all three shifts, the administrator should also:

- Address whether the staffing is posted daily

- Calculate each day to make sure appropriate staff members are present and that you have enough staff budgeted in relation to your current census

PLANNING AND BUDGETING

The following is an example of what I use daily:

Staffing and Census for January 2012

Date	RN	LPN	CNA	Total Nurse Staff
1/01/12	0.52	0.55	2.25	3.61
1/02/12	0.55	0.61	2.51	3.82
1/03/12	0.62	0.60	2.45	3.76
1/04/12	0.65	0.72	2.25	3.75
Average	0.585	0.62	2.365	3.735

Budgeted Based on Census Factor Acuity

<60	0.50	0.55	2.20	3.60
<63	0.53	0.58	2.30	3.65
<67	0.58	0.62	2.40	3.70
<70	0.62	0.65	2.50	3.80

As you can see, each date has a ratio of particular nursing staff to census calculated on a daily basis. On the bottom of the spreadsheet is the budgeted staffing that is set for a certain census interval.

For example, if you have at least 60 but fewer than 63 residents, the budgeted nursing ratios are 0.53 for RNs, 0.58 for LPNs, 2.30 for nursing assistants, and 3.65 for the total nursing staff. I also use other budgeted staff markers, but this will help to provide an example of how budgeting can be numerically based, indicating quantitative information that is not just monetary but also provides important quantitative budgeted staffing information for assessing a facility's goals.

One last thing should be mentioned. Keeping a running tabulation of the month's average for these respective indicators is important. Let's say your census average for the month was 66.51 residents. If you look at the bottom of the budgeted staffing, it gives you a running average. Now let's say that instead of averages for just four days, those averages were complete after the end of the 30-day month. In the staff budgeting information described below, you can look at the numbers of <67 but not less than 63 residents and see how you did for the month. Let us say the RN ratio was 0.60, LPN ratio was 0.61, LNA ratio was 2.35, and total ratio was 3.72. What is evident is that RN and total nurse staffing ratios were slightly higher than budgeted, but the difference was not that great. Overall, staffing for the month was not too low and not excessively high but fell, for the most part, in the budgeted area.

CHAPTER 6

The operating budget

The operating budget is devised for the daily operation of the healthcare facility. The operating budget can usually be subdivided into revenue and expense budgets. Often, these budgets create a fiscal year plan for revenue centers, which are areas of the facility that will generate revenue, and cost or expense centers, which are areas of the facility that will generate expenses. In hospitals, for example, the radiology department can generate both revenue and expenses. The same thing can exist for physical therapy. In long-term care facilities, revenue centers are less prevalent, so managing cost centers is critical. As I already mentioned, managing the staff in a long-term care facility is critical to ensure that your staffing is appropriate based on the census and level of acuity found in your census.

Budgeting is important for setting financial goals, such as estimating increases or decreases in revenue based on inflation, reimbursement reductions, and so forth. However, possibly more important in healthcare than in other industries is managing the healthcare facility's costs or expenses. The budget helps you to do this by giving you a concrete and objective format to examine the respective revenue and cost centers in your facility and to conduct this examination by using variance analysis to determine how much of a variance there is between your actual monthly costs and your budgeted goals. The following example examines one element of the revenue budget and one element of an expense budget and demonstrates the variance analysis that is often used in the analysis process:

Budgeted Revenue			
	OT/PT		Nursing Wages Expense
April 2012 (Budgeted)	$80,000	(Budgeted)	$200,000
Revenue Realized	$81,238.38	Expense Realized	$210,230
Dollar Variance	$1,238.38		($10,230)
Percent Variance	1.547%		5.115%

As shown in the preceding example, the facility met and slightly exceeded its budgeted monthly revenue for the PT/OT department, exceeding the revenue goal by $1,238.38, or 1.547% of the budgeted $80,000 goal established for the month. This is good news. However, examining the expense budget, it was noted that nursing staff wages also exceeded the budgeted expense of $200,000. That was not so good, as the budgeted expense was exceeded by $10,230, or 5.115% of the goal. This is important because any revenue that was

PLANNING AND BUDGETING

incurred could be offset by going over budget. However, one of the important qualities of budgets and budget analysis is that by examining the respective revenue and, especially, cost centers assiduously, the administrator will be able to address problems quickly, before any issues move toward further uncontrolled costs.

In examining the preceding example, the administrator should address:

- Why the expenses were higher

- Whether the higher expenses were needed and justified

- What he or she can control to bring expenses back down to the budgeted level

The capital budget

As mentioned previously, many types of capital, such as equipment that is important for providing healthcare, depreciate, and the useful life of capital runs its course over a number of years. Healthcare facilities, regardless of the type, must be able to address these possible expenses as part of the budget for the next fiscal year. For example, a hospital usually will have a far more extensive capital budget than a long-term care facility, dealing with possible allocations needed for a new specialty hospital unit, CT and MRI equipment that must be obtained, and replacing older EKG and EEG machines with newer and better-quality diagnostic tools.

However, long-term care facilities also must address capital needs and therefore set capital budgets yearly to address these needs. For example, they may have to invest in new parallel bars for therapy, add a new air conditioning system to the facility, and target two new lifts to aid in moving patients with mobility issues, as well as numerous other capital issues that may need to be addressed. Although these capital issues are not as intensive as those found in a hospital environment, they are nonetheless important issues that need to be addressed so that the facility can continue to provide quality care.

Capital budgeting relies on the astute forecasting abilities of the administrator and the administrator's healthcare team. Whether it is for a large hospital or a small, 50-bed nursing facility, capital budgeting relies on the team of individuals informing the administrator about future capital needs. One of the major mistakes made in administration is not looking into the future and failing to adequately forecast one's needs. Therefore, when a CT scanner breaks down, parallel bars collapse due to excessive wear, or an air conditioning system falters due to its age and inability to respond to the demands made upon it, the healthcare facility can find itself in a crisis situation.

CHAPTER 6

Forecasting Capital

As with any business, forecasting the capital needs of a healthcare facility must be done annually and developed into a capital budget to be addressed in the forthcoming fiscal year. Many long-term care facilities often wait and address capital issues as they come along. As I mentioned, this can be disastrous.

Furthermore, just like any other budget, the capital budget should target certain areas as well as estimate a cost and time period during which the capital expenditure will take place. For example, given the preceding examples, you may have to prioritize your capital expenditures based on need and the amount of working capital that is projected to be available to your facility. If your fiscal year starts January 1, your first priority may be to obtain the parallel bars and the two lifts in January. Historically, your facility's greatest level of revenue has been from April to July. Because putting in the new air conditioning unit will be a very large capital expense, which by your well-investigated estimate will cost approximately $300,000 and will take two weeks to install at your facility, your target date for this project may be set during the last two weeks of April or first few weeks of May, when you will not have to deal with heating issues for the building and when the outside temperatures will also not be too hot.

Furthermore, your largest revenue typically happens during this period, and this will aid in having the appropriate amount of liquidity available to address this greater expense.

7 Cost Containment in Long-Term Care

In an era in which reimbursement has become increasingly sparse, cost containment is of major importance for nursing home administrators. However, cost controls are not exclusively the purview of administrators. All administrative staff members should be mindful of the importance of cost control. This does not mean that administration should develop budgets that are so austere that they impinge upon providing good, sound, quality care. But management, and especially the nursing home administrator, has to make sure that superfluous costs are eliminated.

Furthermore, administrators do not have to be accountants or financial experts to employ adequate cost containment measures. Much of the cost control that is used is not so sophisticated that one has to have mastered cost accounting to achieve the goals of the facility. Before moving forward, let's examine the different types of costs that are often mentioned.

Types of Costs

Costs are those things that are incurred against your revenue. They take away from profit and have a negative impact on the bottom line. However, all businesses have costs, and it is important to understand the types of cost that are impacting your long-term care environment.

Fixed costs

Fixed costs do not vary or change. In long-term care, fixed costs do not change with the level of census or resident need. For example, building lease or rental agreements and utilities still have to be paid regardless of the census in the building. Furthermore, regardless of the census, a building must have a full-time administrator and director of nursing.

Variable costs

Variable costs, on the other hand, fluctuate directly with productive activity and the census of the building. For example, the number of nursing care personnel needed is a variable cost. The number of nursing care personnel will vary directly when the census is 50 rather than 100. Food costs are also variable.

Semivariable costs

Semivariable costs sit in the middle of fixed and variable costs; they vary not so much due to census as due to the management decisions regarding these costs. For example, advertisement cost would be a semivariable cost that is not totally dependent upon the census yet is often set by the administrator.

Direct and indirect costs

Direct costs are specially directed to a service or product. For example, purchasing equipment for the facility to assist in maintenance is a direct cost to the maintenance department. The cost of your administrator and nursing administrative staff is a direct labor cost.

Indirect costs are not directly or easily placed into a specific department and may lead to costs in more than one area. For example, absenteeism and turnover are indirect costs that affect labor costs, training, and recruiting. Often, indirect costs are more insidious because they are not as clear cut or easily identifiable.

Overhead costs

One type of cost most people have heard of is *overhead cost*, or the cost of running a business. All businesses have a level of overhead, but excessive overhead costs can be extremely detrimental to a business. Acute care hospitals often have to deal with many types of overhead costs, especially for expensive equipment such as MRI machines, PET and CAT scanners, and so forth. In this type of situation, the demand is often created to attempt to deal with and overset the overhead costs.

Long-term care facilities do not have as many of these capital items to create the same degree of overhead. However, they do have to be aware of avoiding the excessive overhead costs related to running a nursing care facility. For example, excessive inventory buildup or using equipment that may not be used very often can be quite expensive to nursing homes.

COST CONTAINMENT IN LONG-TERM CARE

Period costs

Period costs are costs allocated over a particular period and are contrasted with point costs, which reflect a cost on a particular occasion. Some period costs cannot be avoided, such as building rental or lease fees paid during the month. Having too many rentals or lease fees creates an excessive period cost that needs to be reduced. If you are renting bariatric beds, for example, and you have a considerable number of bariatric residents, it is probably wiser to purchase the beds, reducing your rental costs; if you have a good bariatric clientele, the payback period will probably be quite short.

Sunk costs

If you purchase something, regardless of whether it was a wise purchase or investment, your cost is sunk in the purchase of this equipment. If the equipment, items, and so on are purchased and used and they do not work out, the cost is a *sunk cost*. This is similar to purchasing a stock and losing money. You have a sunk cost.

Opportunity costs

When you forego one activity and choose another, this is often referred to as an *opportunity cost*. It is the cost you incur by not choosing the alternative. For example, say your resources are limited. If you need equipment X and Y but you have enough money to purchase only equipment X, the opportunity cost you incurred was your inability to purchase equipment Y at the expense of purchasing equipment X. Because facilities have only a finite amount of financial resources by purchasing more of equipment X, you have less you can spend on equipment Y. This is the opportunity cost for equipment Y due to the purchase invested in equipment X.

Intangible costs

Intangible costs are difficult to quantify and measure. The reputation of your facility, goodwill, and trade names are often intangible resources, and intangible costs can affect them as well. If your facility has traditionally had a good reputation and suddenly it has a bad survey, this can incur a large intangible cost on the facility's reputation. However, because intangible costs are difficult to measure, their material effect is not as directly measurable as other costs.

CHAPTER 7

Necessary and unnecessary costs

Finally, you can make a distinction between necessary and unnecessary costs. *Necessary costs* are necessary and lead to an increase in profits for the facility. Conversely, *unnecessary costs* are costs which, when eliminated, help to increase the facility's profit margin. Thus, this becomes a critical distinction for administrators to examine. Is the cost necessary, leading to better care and, with it, profit? Or is it a superfluous, unnecessary cost, that, if eliminated, will enhance the facility's profit margin? Many critical decisions administrators make revolve around the problem of necessary versus unnecessary costs.

8 PPDs as the Benchmark for Measurement

Determining PPD

The standard administrators use most commonly in long-term care, especially in measuring costs in relation to the patient, is the per patient day (PPD) standard. This is a budgeted measure based on hours per patient day (HPPD) or dollars per patient day (DPPD). Nursing home administrators will often look at the PPD in hours or dollars as it relates to the patient census to provide a more accurate and detailed understanding of where they stand in their daily budget. This especially becomes a powerful tool for managing costs daily. To provide an example of its importance, a nursing home may be under its budget in employee salaries for the month by $20,000. Yet because it was well below its average daily census for the month, it was actually over budget on the PPDs for employee salaries. What does this tell us? It tells us that even though on an aggregate level our dollars were below budget, we were still spending too much money on salaries given the number of residents that we had in the building. Therefore, because this is such an important area for long-term care administrators to understand, it behooves us to examine it in closer detail.

Scenario 1

For example, let's say that on a daily basis in your facility you set an HPPD of 3.02 for nursing care provided to your residents. This will often include the total number of hours in a 24-hour period for nurse assistants and nurses that provide direct nursing care. Now let's say that you set your HPPD budget at 3.02 for nursing care. You have a 200-bed facility, but at the current time only 150 beds are occupied. You would calculate the number of nursing hours (nurse assistants plus nurses who provide direct care) as such:

$3.02 \times 150 = 453$ nursing hours for a 24-hour period to stay within the HPPD of 3.02

CHAPTER 8

If you divide 453 by 8, which is the standard number of hours that most personnel work per shift, this equals 56.625. This means that roughly 56 to 57 nursing personnel providing direct care should exist for a 24-hour period to stay close to the 3.02 HPPD budget.

Scenario 2

Now let's say that as the administrator, you examine your daily staffing report and you notice that you have 520 direct care nursing hours for a 24-hour period and your census is 150. In doing the math, you divide 150 into 520 and determine that your HPPD is 3.46. It does not seem like much, but apparent small deviations in PPD often equal large unnecessary costs. In reality, a 0.44 PPD variance from the budget is a large variance, and most seasoned administrators recognize this quickly.

Scenario 3

As mentioned, you also can determine PPD on the basis of dollars. Most people will use the HPPD mentioned previously on a daily basis because it is often quicker to produce and it is quicker to introduce cost control with this information. However, month-end financial statements often like to use DPPD. For example, let's say that your total revenue generated during the month was $953,000 and your expenses were $720,000. In your 200-bed facility, your daily average census equals 187.38 residents. You calculated this by dividing the total number of resident days by the number of days in the month. An average daily census for the month of 187.38 divided by 200 gives you a 93.69% occupancy rate. In this scenario, your revenue exceeds your expenses by $233,000. If you multiply 187.38 by 31, you get the number of total patient days in your facility for the month, which, when rounded off, is 5,809 days. If you divide the number of days by the total revenue, you get a DPPD of $164.05 for revenue. If you divide the total expenses by the total resident days, you obtain a DPPD of $123.95 for expenses.

Scenario 4

Let's say your budgeted revenue PPD is $162 and your budgeted expense PPD is $125. In this case, you did fairly well for the month. You exceeded the revenue DPPD and you were under the expenses DPPD. That is pretty much where you would like to be.

However, what happens when your PPD for hours or expenses runs high? In the scenario where there are 520 direct care nursing hours for a census of 150 on a budgeted HPPD of 3.02, a few things need to happen. The most obvious is that you have to reduce your staff to 3.02 × 150 = 453 hours divided by 8, which means you need 56 to 57 staff members. At 520 hours, you have 65 staff members, and you therefore need to reduce at least eight full-time eight-hour staff members for the day to get close to your budget.

You could also admit 22 more residents and reach a census of 172 to meet your budget, but for most nursing homes, 22 admissions in a day is not possible. Also, some months you will not be able to attain your budgeted revenue. Again, in the preceding example, a DPPD of $162 was set for your revenue, and your expense PPD was set at $125. What if your revenue PPD for the month was $157? It becomes even more important to watch your expenses in this case. If you go well above your expense PPD, it can be problematic and costly to the facility. But if you reduce your expenses slightly as well or stay close to your stated DPPD for expenses, you minimize any financial problems.

PPD and the Entire Facility

It is important to understand that one must also keep tabs on the PPDs within individual areas. The PPDs for not just nursing but also rehabilitation, the kitchen, housekeeping, laundry, and maintenance are usually the major areas that need to be examined daily for proper staffing.

However, although many of these areas are variable or semivariable costs, some costs can be fixed and not as amenable to examining through daily PPDs. Also, although keeping tabs on your budget through your PPDs is census driven for the most part, an administrator cannot just focus purely on the head count in the building. In fact, doing so leads to a bottom-line bean counter looking just at dollars and cents and failing to take the larger needs of the facility into consideration, and this is plain stupid. You must always structure your budget and your staffing needs based on the acuity of the facility. Therefore, you must develop a new budget based on your anticipated acuity for the year and examine your daily PPDs in the context of your current daily acuity.

Looking at the bigger picture

Context is an important word. Many administrators are so driven by numbers that they fail to see the larger picture of their facility. Administrators as well as other administrative staff members have to be concerned with the budgetary numbers on a daily basis to maintain a properly running facility. But you also have to be aware of the context of care that is in your facility during any given day. A resident may need 1:1 monitoring, requiring an extra staff member on each shift. In this case, paying attention to the pure bottom line could severely compromise the care that is rendered, not only to this one resident but also to other residents as well.

CHAPTER 8

The financial efficiency of a facility is important, but it should never compromise the care and safety of the residents it services. Therefore, when developing a budget for the year, you must consider the number of staff members at each level of the census required to provide optimal care and safety and review this on a daily basis. Frankly, sometimes, especially during an unanticipated heightened acuity, you must deviate from your budget to service your residents with the best possible quality.

Monitoring Costs Through Spend-Downs

As mentioned earlier, cost control is important for all administrative staff members. One of the easiest ways to have other staff members involved in cost control and containment is to develop spend-down sheets for each department, especially dealing with supply costs. The department heads should complete these spend-down sheets each month and review them at the end of each month with the administrator.

Completing a spend-down sheet

Spend-down sheets are easy to use and complete. You begin with a specific budgeted amount for the month and subtract the amount of each expenditure from the previous balance, as you would do with your own checkbook. Spend-down sheets are nice because they are easy for staff members to use. However, for spend-down sheets to be a successful budgeting control tool, department managers must use them assiduously, making sure that every expenditure that needs to be accounted for is placed in the spend-down sheet for that month.

One of the largest errors made with the spend-down sheets is that department managers will just enter the expense and not total the column. This is the same mistake people make with their checkbooks, and when they finally total the amount they find they are excessively overdrawn. This is why anyone using a spend-down sheet needs to know that he or she must calculate the new balance after each expense is placed on the form. Otherwise, the spend-down sheet becomes a useless tool. Spend-down sheets are meant to focus cost control on each cost that is incurred, when it is incurred. Only by doing this can you use spend-down sheets effectively.

9 Labor Costs

Labor costs is a large area that needs to be controlled constantly. As mentioned earlier in this book, you must examine labor costs daily to ensure that optimal staffing is available to address resident needs and that staffing is not excessive. One of the most common ways of examining labor costs is to use the hour per patient day (HPPD) formula.

However, as noted earlier, the administrator must also monitor acuity on a daily basis and ensure that proper staffing fits not only the number of residents but also the acuity level. That being said, salaries and benefits often create about 60% of the total expenses in long-term care facilities, and because healthcare, and especially long-term care, is so labor-intensive, staffing costs are imperative for proper cost management.

What to Look For

You must examine a few different things in the area of labor costs. First, you must examine the number of labor hours needed each day and the productivity of your workers. The first way you can examine the number of labor hours and associated costs is to determine how many full-time equivalent (FTE) workers you need each day. For example, if for 120 residents you need 357 labor hours in nursing to provide optimal care, you would calculate the number of labor hours needed as follows:

$$\frac{357}{8} = 44.625 \text{ FTEs}$$

This means that for a census of 120 residents at the budgeted labor hours, you need approximately 45 nursing care staff members.

CHAPTER 9

Worker productivity is also important. Are your workers productive, and if so, to what level? Productivity is often used to measure the utilization of workers. You can measure productivity as follows:

$$\text{Productivity} = \frac{\text{Required Staff}}{\text{Provided Staff}} \times 100$$

For 100% productivity, the required staff should match the provided staff. If the provided staff is far in excess of the required staff, productivity will go down. If the provided staff is far below what is required, your productivity may be too high to the point where you are burning out your employees.

Furthermore, regarding productivity, Jacobs (1986) states that a 15% variance is acceptable per day and a 10% variance is acceptable if it is calculated on a weekly basis. Therefore, on a daily basis, 100% plus or minus the suggested variance is pretty much the benchmark for productivity. Thus, a variance of less than 15% is not achieving optimal worker productivity, and a variance that is higher than 15% may be creating a very tired, burned-out workforce.

Generally speaking, productivity is the ratio of the output of goods and services to the input invested into such activity (e.g., worker hours). For example, if you have a nursing unit of 50 residents and have six certified nursing assistants (CNA) working the same eight-hour shift to provide nursing care to the residents, the productivity of each of the six workers can be determined as follows:

$$\text{Productivity} = \frac{50 \text{ residents}}{6 \text{ certified nurse assistants}} = 8.33$$

According to this equation, each CNA is servicing statistically 8.33 residents. Given the 50 residents, what would happen if the number of CNAs is reduced to five per eight-hour shift? The productivity equation appears as follows:

$$\text{Productivity} = \frac{50 \text{ residents}}{5 \text{ certified nurse assistants}} = 10$$

LABOR COSTS

The second equation actually reflects increased worker productivity, if the five CNAs are able to provide care and complete their work in the same eight-hour time period as the six CNAs were able to do. The second equation now demonstrates that five CNAs can provide and complete care for all 50 residents within an eight-hour shift, and each CNA can increase his or her productivity to statistically 10 residents as opposed to 8.33 residents.

This is not the only factor that has to be examined when calculating productivity. Cost accountants are going to be concerned with changes in the "unit labor costs." The unit labor cost is equal to hourly compensation divided by productivity (United States Department of Labor).

$$\text{Unit labor costs} = \frac{\text{Hourly compensation}}{\text{Productivity}}$$

To understand how the unit labor cost relates to productivity, consider the following scenarios.

Scenario one: There is a unit of 50 residents. There are six CNAs caring for the 50 residents during an eight-hour shift. Each CNA earns $12 per hour. The following is the calculation:

> $12 per hour x 8 hours worked x 6 certified nurse assistants = $576
> Divide this by 50 residents: 576/50 = $11.52 of worker pay per resident

Scenario two: There is a unit of 50 residents. However, now there are only five CNAs caring for the 50 residents during an eight-hour shift. Each CNA earns $12 per hour. The following is the calculation:

> $12 per hour x 8 hours worked x 5 certified nurse assistants = $480
> Divide this by 50 residents: 480/5 = $9.60 of worker pay per resident

In the first scenario, the unit cost was $11.52 per resident for the eight-hour shift. In the second scenario, the unit cost was considerably less, at $9.60 per resident. Therefore, if the same amount of work was able to be achieved in the second scenario as in the first scenario, this would show that on a cost accounting basis, using five nurse assistants is more productive, especially financially, for the healthcare facility.

CHAPTER 9

However, productivity is a measure of quantity, and it does not necessarily equate with quality. The ability to obtain the greatest productivity and efficiency from each dollar invested in your operational environment is paramount, and this mantra is not just applicable for healthcare management but for all forms of operational management. The administrator needs to align productivity with quality in care to achieve an optimal result in care. There is often no hard and fast rule of where to draw the line. Therefore, the healthcare administrator has to understand where he or she is getting the best productivity financially, while still providing high-level care. By streamlining staff, subsequently reducing the unit cost and apparently enhancing productivity numbers, without looking at other areas, the productivity measures are not really measuring anything but an administrator's attempt to reduce costs at the expense of care.

Overtime and Pool Use

Overtime as well as reliance on nursing pools is another critical area that facility administrators must address. Many facilities rely too heavily on nursing pools. You should view nursing pools as a last-ditch effort to obtain needed staff members. First, nursing pools are expensive because their salaries are high and incentives are provided to achieve profits. Furthermore, although those who staff nursing pools are qualified, hiring staff members from the outside takes away from the continuity that must exist to continue providing excellent nursing care.

Most nursing pool staff members have to orient themselves to your facility, and most do not know the residents, families, and other staff members who provide continuity in care. Moreover, nursing pool staff members are often not vested in your facility with the same commitment that other permanent staff members have, and this is a major problem. Thus, sometimes nursing pool staff may be needed, but you should use them as a last resort. It is better to cultivate a good working climate that attracts and keeps workers so that you do not need to turn to nursing pools.

Overtime is an inevitable issue in healthcare. It is almost impossible to totally eliminate all overtime, especially in the patient care area. However, when overtime becomes a runaway expense, you need to bring it into check quickly. Generally speaking, the industry rate of overtime in long-term care runs between 3% and 5%.

For sure, lower than 3% is great if you can still maintain optimal staffing. However, as your labor cost for overtime extends beyond 5%, you must keep a cautious eye on preventing it from escalating and being part of the regular daily regime.

LABOR COSTS

If you continue to run high overtime rates, this is a sign that your scheduling is not being closely monitored or you have a chronic staff shortage that is a symptom of other facility labor problems (e.g., wages, benefits, work conditions, etc.) that you must scrutinize closely. For example, many facilities balk at raising their wages to attract more workers, and yet they will continue to maintain a wage problem and pay exorbitant payroll expenses in overtime. Although the increase in wages may add $10,000 more to the payroll, this is far better than paying out two or three times that in overtime.

Absenteeism

As a cost control issue, high absentee rates lead to the need for overtime and nursing pool use. Also, absenteeism by certain employees leads to greater stress for the workers who must cover for those who are absent.

When absenteeism is excessive, it leads to disenchantment among consistently good employees, anger toward employees who do not carry their weight, and disenchantment with the facility if it continues to let the excessive absentee rate continue without punishment. Therefore, as you can see, excessive absenteeism not only leads to financial problems for the facility, but it also leads to demoralization within the work environment.

Therefore, it is necessary to be aware of your absentee rate. It is a sign of the psychological and social health of your labor force, which, if not corrected, can lead to runaway costs. Although the administrator does not have to do this, the scheduler should be able to provide information and track this information on a daily, weekly, and monthly basis. The following is how you calculate the absentee rate:

$$\text{Daily Absentee Rate} = \frac{\text{Number of Absences for the Day}}{\text{Number of Employees Scheduled}} \times 100$$

$$\text{Monthly Absentee Rate} = \frac{\text{Number of Absent Days for the Month}}{\text{Total Employees} \times \text{Days in Month}} \times 100$$

In the long-term care industry, 2.5% is often viewed as an acceptable standard of absenteeism for the month (Jacobs 1986). Anything higher than that level can indicate worker dissatisfaction and a work culture that is not addressing many of the needs that workers have for coming to work consistently.

CHAPTER 9

You must deal with excessive absenteeism quickly and uniformly. During certain periods, such as the flu season, absentee rates may increase, but when they are consistently high, you must address this cost issue on a human resource level. Providing consistent discipline for excessive absenteeism is important, as is ensuring that the discipline is carried out in a uniform manner.

Solutions to absenteeism

Enhancing the work culture and being receptive to employees' complaints can help to solve the problem of absenteeism. For certain days, such as weekends, you could introduce a policy that will discourage absenteeism, such as makeup days on the following weekends. Hire employees with good track records, using references as checks. And encourage other workers to support the attendance policy, rewarding them for good attendance and creating worker empowerment to allow them to place pressure on their working peers. In fact, workers are often the best source of keeping noncompliant workers in line. Finally, do not keep giving second chances to those who have attendance problems. Remember, you must address this issue equally and succinctly.

Turnover

As anyone who has worked in long-term care can attest, the work is hard and often the pay is far from exorbitant. Therefore, it is important to attempt to select workers who will stay at your facility.

This is easier said than done, and there is no great science that provides certainty in your recruitment. However, cursory interviews and jumping at the first candidate should be cautioned against, because this difficulty typically leads to higher turnover without adequately screening your recruits. Data show that turnover among most new employees typically occurs within the first 90 days of employment. Therefore, having a structured recruitment process, if done correctly, can prevent you from hiring the wrong employees.

Furthermore, typically a facility will invest a few thousand dollars in an employee's training and recruitment. When that employee leaves quickly, the facility also faces a cost in this area.

A certain level of turnover is viewed as acceptable in long-term care. In nursing homes, turnover often reaches high levels, with many facilities experiencing turnover rates that are well over 50% annually in certain areas, and in some departments the annual turnover may well approach, or even exceed, 100%. Because of the need to train new employees, expenses associated with recruitment costs, and calling upon overtime staff members to fill in for those who have left or have been terminated, it becomes obvious that turnover can be a major cost that needs to be controlled.

LABOR COSTS

Turnover rate, stability rate, and average length of employment rate

Three equations are of interest for understanding the stability of your workforce: the turnover rate, the stability rate, and the average length of employment rate (Jacobs 1986). All three provide a good understanding of your workforce, its culture, and problems that may exist.

You can calculate the *turnover rate* as follows:

$$\text{Turnover Rate} = \frac{\text{Number of Terminations (Forced or Unforced)}}{\text{Number of Employees}} \times 100$$

Examining this monthly will help you quickly see whether there are any problems, and it will show you what it is costing your facility to train new workers. Many companies are attempting to keep their annual turnover rates at less than 50%, and in this industry, that is hard to do. However, the lower the turnover rate, generally the greater the workforce stability and continuity.

You also can examine your facility's level of stability through its *stability rate*. The stability rate looks at the rate of employees who start employment and are still around after one month. However, you can also extend this to larger time periods, such as looking at the number of employees still employed after 90 days or more. The following is the equation to use:

$$\text{Daily Absentee Rate} = \frac{\text{Number of Beginning Employees Remaining (From Start, to 30, 60, 90 Days, etc.)}}{\text{Number of Employees at the Beginning}} \times 100$$

For example, if 22 new employees start working at your facility April 1, on April 30 you could determine the one-month worker stability rate. If at the end of the month 17 employees still were employed, the equation would look as follows:

$$\text{Stability Rate} = \frac{17}{22} \times 100 = 77.27\%$$

CHAPTER 9

At first glance, you may think this is the same as the turnover rate. But the percentage states that 77.27% of your new workforce did not turn over, and at the same time your total turnover was associated with 22.73% of your positions in the company (Jacobs 1986). Therefore, a small number of positions at your facility are accounting for most of the turnover.

Another important statistic that provides a large amount of information about your work culture is the average length of employment rate. In fact, this can be useful for helping to market your facility if the average length of employment is high. As you can imagine, if average length of employment is low, often worker instability exists and the cost extends not only to training and recruitment but also to the care that one provides.

Higher average length of employment often is associated with greater workforce continuity, which in turn impacts the quality of care that is provided. Many prospective consumers looking for placement of a loved one are too often taken in by the aesthetics of the facility when critical questions they should ask are what the facility's turnover rate is and what the facility's average length of employment rate is.

The average length of employment is calculated as follows:

$$\text{Average Length of Employment} = \frac{\text{Sum of Length of Service for All Employees}}{\text{Total Number of Employees}}$$

As an example, let's say you have 10 employees (a low number for a nursing home, but good for an example). The employees' lengths of service, in years, are 5.8, 2.1, 2.5, 0.5, 9.7, 15.2, 22.5, 2.3, 1.2, and 15.5, for a total of 77.3 years.

$$\frac{77.3}{10} = 7.73 \text{ Years of Average Employment}$$

That is not bad as far as average years of employment is concerned. However, you must also notice that extremes in both the high and low ranges can impact the average.

10 The Staff

The Dietary Department

A facility's staffing needs to be sufficient to address the census in the building as well as its specific dietary needs. Many individuals like to budget this area based on staff hours worked and determine the average number of meals that are served based on hours worked. It is commonly assumed that an average of seven to eight meals are served per hour worked. This does not mean that meals are served constantly; it is an average. For example, using this type of process to create a budget for a dietary staff, if you have a facility housing 100 residents, 100 × 3 meals per day divided by the constant of 7 equals 42.86 hours of dietary staff needed each day.

The preceding method does not provide much latitude for addressing other issues that may come up as part of the dietary issues that are faced. Therefore, a better way is often to set a budget, based on per patient day (PPD), which also varies with the census that the facility has to serve. The dietary manager will have to examine the staffing daily in accordance with the census, as well as the needs of the facility.

Food

A major dietary area you should scrutinize closely is food costs—in particular, raw food costs. This is another area where use of a spend-down sheet can be valuable.

For example, if your raw food PPD is $3.50 × days in the month (31) × the budgeted census of 112, you would set your spend-down with a starting budgeted total for the month at $12,152. Raw food is a big expense, because it makes up most of a facility's food budget. Moreover, it can become a runaway expense if you do not monitor it closely. Also, your budget should provide for a pleasant dining experience; however, daily T-bone steaks will probably not fit into your budget. Also monitor your vendors in this area. Some vendors are more expensive than others and sometimes the more expensive vendors have poorer food quality.

CHAPTER 10

Supplies

Dietary supplies are another area that needs to be closely examined, along with house formulas and special thickening solutions and kitchen cleaning chemicals. Again, using the same PPD budgeted formula and spend-down sheet as demonstrated earlier in these areas for supplies, formulas, thickening solutions, and cleaning chemicals will help keep the kitchen on budget. Most facilities are running between $4 to $5 for resident PPD dietary needs. If this runs too low, it may indicate that you do not provide a pleasurable dining experience. Conversely, if it runs too high, it may indicate that you are ordering excessively or that your provisions are becoming too exorbitant.

The Housekeeping Department

There are no mandated numerical requirements for staffing other than providing housekeeping services that are appropriate to address the needs of the facility. However, generally there is a rule of thumb that states that there should be approximately one eight-hour staff member for every 1,000 square feet in the building. That being said, many individuals often establish housekeeping as a fixed cost (e.g., there will be 40 hours of housekeeping regardless of the census). Here again, you must determine housekeeping needs based on such factors as the size and age of the building, the mobility and acuity of your residents, and so forth. You determine the productivity ratio to ensure that you are getting appropriate productivity from your staff. Furthermore, although this is an area that is often minimized to reduce costs incurred, having a staff that is able to address all the housekeeping concerns of the building is important.

Floor care

Frequently, floor care is part of housekeeping and is included in the housekeeping budget. There is no problem with this, as long as the budget was established to accommodate floor care. I recommend that floor care personnel be budgeted into the daily census. There are a couple reasons for this. One is that daily floor care is important for demonstrating the cleanliness of a facility. Many people who come into your building quickly gravitate to the floors as an indicator of cleanliness. Second, a skilled floor care person who is efficient at waxing, stripping, and general floor maintenance can save money in the long run.

Housekeeping personnel

It is important to establish the optimal number of housekeeping personnel as a necessary cost. Moreover, inadequate housekeeping leads to costs paid out in poor surveys and civil monetary penalties, and the

THE STAFF

intangible costs for marketing and consumer recognition for a facility can be high if you try to minimize this area. A facility, regardless of age, should present itself as clean and accommodating. If you reduce your staff to the point where floor care is being provided infrequently, and other areas cannot be targeted due to inadequate staffing levels, you need to obtain additional staff members. If staffing is excessive, your productivity rate will decline and people will have too much empty time on their hands. Again, as the administrator, you must determine the optimal level of housekeepers in your facility to accommodate your needs in this area.

The housekeeping supervisor also must monitor the supplies that are used through spend-down sheets developed on a monthly budgeted level by the administrator. Important supplies that must be monitored through spend-downs are chemical agents and supplies such as garbage bags and paper towels. In addition, these supplies need to be inventoried because housekeeping supplies are a major source of theft inside facilities. They must be stored in a locked area with limited access to provide the necessary internal control for inventory.

The housekeeping supervisor and administrator should often attempt to look at other vendors for price comparisons. Many vendors can provide the same or similar quality cleaning products at a lower price. Moreover, mixing cleaning solutions often leads to waste through excessive chemical use. Therefore, it is often better to get a cleaning solution that offers you a dispenser that provides the appropriate solute/solution concentration. This in itself can save a great deal of cost. Also, although many people will attempt to save money by buying cheaper products, and this may be justified, some products are cheap because of their poor quality, resulting in cost escalation in the long run.

The Laundry Department

Laundry is another area that has to be adjusted to meet the facility's linen demands. Once again, there are no clear numerical rules on how many workers are needed in this area, but there are some general guidelines. The department's productivity is often centered on the following rule of thumb: one work hour for every 100 pounds of laundry. Therefore, if your facility launders approximately 1,600 pounds of laundry each day, you should have approximately two full-time, eight-hour laundry personnel each day.

Staff

You need to examine how you schedule your laundry personnel. Laundry does not have to be a 24-hour operation, as it can often lead to low productivity rates among laundry personnel on the midnight shift.

Conversely, running one shift may lead to increased productivity but also an excessive and unreasonable burden on the staff that is attempting to play catch-up from the afternoon and midnight shifts. Therefore, it is often prudent to make the laundry duties expand over a period of at least 12–16 hours. In this way, you have covered the laundering that needs to be completed at an optimal level, without having to relegate excessive catch-up duties to those who first come in on the morning shift.

Supplies

Laundry chemicals used and purchased, similar to housekeeping, can be monitored through a monthly spend-down budget. Naturally, excessive use of chemicals leads to heightened costs. Metered mixtures that can be attached to washing machines often provide a good means of cost savings in this area by not over-using chemical agents. Furthermore, it is important to ensure that the washers and dryers are cleaned and that lint screens are cleaned regularly throughout the day. Machines that are not running at an optimal level will lead to rewashing, and this rework adds to increasing costs.

Load amount

The amount of laundry placed into a washing machine also influences cost. If too little is being placed in the washing machine, the cost you are incurring for using cleaning chemicals and work hours will increase. Jacobs (1986) states that the PPD for laundry weight is approximately 8–10 pounds PPD for most nursing care facilities. Therefore, if yours is a 150-bed facility with a laundry weight PPD of 10 pounds, you have a budgeted daily laundry PPD of 1,500 pounds, or 46,500 pounds for the month. This is running roughly two full-time laundry staff members per day. Failing to optimize the amount that can be placed into a washer and dryer increases the cost of a facility's laundry expenses. Further, while machines are running, the laundry staff should also be involved in folding, sorting, and delivering the laundry. There should be no large intervals where the laundry staff members are doing nothing.

Linen costs

Costs for laundry are also increased by linen needs. Temperatures need to be followed to provide infection control; however, excessive temperatures lead to degradation of linens. Use of chemicals that are too harsh can cause the same problem. These will cause early and unnecessary replacement costs.

Another major cost is incurred when linens are thrown away due to worker laziness. Soiled linen needs to be rinsed in the hopper and placed in appropriately marked bags. However, a major expense in nursing homes occurs when washed clothes and towels are thrown away just because they are soiled. First, staff members should be made aware of the cost of this type of activity. When a person is found to be doing this, he or she should be disciplined. Furthermore, addressing residents' needs promptly and toileting them as needed can often forestall messes on towels, washcloths, and bed sheets. In addition, linen should be obtained only as needed from the clean linen storage area. Hoarding linen to carry and do rounds with often leads to it being misplaced or thrown out, not to mention that it is an infection control issue.

The Maintenance Staff

Hiring qualified maintenance personnel can reduce costs at a facility. One of the major mistakes many people make is hiring a "handyman" to handle everything. A maintenance person should have a thorough knowledge of electrical, machinery maintenance, plumbing, plant restoration, and, in general, just about everything that it takes to maintain and fix issues that crop up daily within a facility.

Hiring a person who has a broad background in many of these areas will save your facility money. This does not mean this person must be an expert in all these areas, but it does mean he or she needs to have a broad working knowledge of plant maintenance so that you do not have to also hire outside help.

Preventive maintenance

Important to maintaining a sound cost control program is having a good preventive maintenance program. Here again, having a person or persons who are skilled in the area and understand the importance of preventive maintenance toward enhancing the longevity of the facility and reducing the likelihood for major problems that are exacerbated due to poor preventive oversight saves money and reduces costs. A good preventive maintenance person can reduce costs through his or her experience and be able to predict where problems will exist and how to preclude issues from happening, hence leading to unnecessary costs.

Should we hire more than one?

How many maintenance personnel are needed? This depends on the size and age of the building. In small buildings with a census of less than 100, you may be able to get by with one full-time staff member. However, in buildings that are larger and older, you probably will need at least two full-time maintenance personnel. If the building is older and needs a considerable level of maintenance work, such as ceiling tile replacement and painting, you may want to budget for a project maintenance person who is strictly dedicated to doing this type of work.

CHAPTER 10

Good maintenance personnel who are experienced—especially in dealing with healthcare and long-term care facilities—can save you money in other areas as well. For example, they can often head up the safety committee and be the administrator's key right-hand person in preventing Occupational Safety and Health Administration and life safety citations. Many good maintenance personnel who have been employed in the long-term care arena know a considerable amount about survey preparation and the regulatory environment. Therefore, you should base your choice of lead maintenance personnel on how they can help you reduce costs through their knowledge of plant operations, preventive maintenance, and the regulatory environment.

11 Medicaid, Medicare, and Third-Party Payment

Medicaid

Medicaid is the dominant source of finances for the nursing home industry, with an estimated 70% of all nursing home income coming from Medicaid reimbursement (Davis, Haacker, & Townsend, 2002). Medicaid holds less weight in the acute care area as a source of funding. Medicaid was initially set up as a health insurance option for those who are indigent, and this continues to be its main purpose, regardless of age. However, older adults who need extensive long-term care often exhaust their financial resources, leaving them dependent on Medicaid to pay their nursing home bills due to their level of indigence.

Established as Title XIX of the Social Security Act under President Johnson's administration as part of his "war on poverty" legislation, Medicaid was targeted to assist the indigent, many of whom were not receiving any form of healthcare. However, it also has become an impetus for the nursing home industry, giving many residents who have exhausted their resources a way to pay for continued care within a nursing home environment.

Medicaid is a public assistance program to which the federal and state governments contribute. Usually the state contributes funds equal to those contributed by the federal government. Nevertheless, the federal government allows the state to establish eligibility requirements for Medicaid. The eligibility requirements established are for all ages and not just the elderly, yet states do establish the criteria that are needed for older adults to receive Medicaid funding for nursing home care.

Usually, Medicaid is a form of reimbursement of last resort, and it will be initiated only after a resident has exhausted any Medicare, private insurance, and private pay expenses available to him or her. Therefore, before Medicaid can go into effect, each state usually establishes requirements in which a

CHAPTER 11

considerable level of a resident's personal assets are exhausted before the resident is eligible for nursing home reimbursement.

The administrator must be cognizant of those residents who become established under Medicaid and those who are left pending. Certain states may overlook or not act on certain individuals that have been submitted for Medicaid approval. Too many residents with cases that have not been acted on promptly and remain as pending can be a financial hardship to your facility.

Medicaid and internal accounting

It is important that the necessary internal accounting for Medicaid funds be handled appropriately and when the funds are received. State source documents related to Medicaid disbursement should be kept on file. The state will usually expect your accountants to conduct a yearly reconciliation of the facility's Medicaid funds, and, therefore, the accountants often rely on the documentation you have available. This documentation needs to be accurate and must account for all the financial reimbursement made to your facility during a given fiscal year.

It is imperative that you and your bookkeeper ensure that each reimbursement is consistent with the reimbursement the state has deemed appropriate for each resident. Catching mistakes quickly can prevent you from having to pay money back to the state that you should not have received when the reconciliation report is filed. It can also address mistakes made by the state if the state has not disbursed adequate funds consistent with what it was supposed to allocate given each resident.

The Start of a New Era

In the early 1980s, we entered an era of cost containment that was exemplified by the introduction of diagnosis-related groups (DRG). More than 400 diagnostic classifications were made, and specific reimbursement was coded for each diagnostic code under Medicare. For individuals who were hospitalized for a specific condition, a certain amount of money was paid, and if the patient's treatment exceeded the amount that was allocated for the specific diagnostic category, the hospital lost money.

Conversely, if the hospital released the patient and the cost of the patient's care did not exceed the disbursement, the hospital made money. Therefore, hospitals had an incentive to release patients earlier, and even move many services to outpatient settings because DRGs did not carry the same weight in these areas as did inpatient treatment in a hospital setting. This had a profound effect on changing the long-term care setting as well, as many patients being released from hospitals now came to these settings sicker and with a higher level of acuity once reserved only for hospital patients.

Nevertheless, in the early 1980s, the healthcare industry moved from a retrospective reimbursement environment, where the cost of care was reimbursed after the care was rendered, to a prospective reimbursement environment, where a set fee and salary were established and where healthcare facilities and healthcare practitioners had to work within the fiscal parameters that were set for them in the delivery of care (Weiss 2004).

This system is radically different from the traditional fee-for-service or free-enterprise medicine system that had dominated the healthcare landscape in the United States. The profound effect of this new area of cost containment has had an influence not just on the hospital environment but also on the long-term care industry.

Medicare

The Balanced Budget Act of 1997 had a profound effect on reimbursement to nursing facilities, especially through Title XVIII, or Medicare. With this Act, a prospective payment system (PPS) was introduced that used 44 different types of resource utilization groups (RUG) and increased to 53 RUG categories. The most current billing system, updated in October 2010, created a system of 66 categories. Medicare residents in nursing homes were evaluated and, based on the more rigorous criteria of resident evaluations, placed into one of these different billing categories.

Each October, the federal government reevaluates each RUG category and determines the reimbursement amount. The reimbursement amount may be different for the same RUG based on the location of the nursing facility—that is, whether it is in a rural, suburban, or major metropolitan area.

Medicare is an important part of the Social Security Act, and, as mentioned, its focus is almost entirely on providing medical insurance for older adults, with the exception of some younger individuals who may receive support from this provision due to a qualifying disability. Those who are eligible for Social Security benefits become eligible for Medicare at the age of 65.

Medicare Parts A, B, C, and D

Traditionally, Medicare has been available in three forms: Parts A, B, and C. However, the recent passage of Medicare Part D has created prescription coverage for older adults.

CHAPTER 11

Medicare Part A is offered to all individuals age 65 and older, and it provides hospitalization coverage. After paying the first day of coverage, Medicare provides 60 days of hospital coverage. If additional hospital coverage is needed, 30 days will be provided with a coinsurance fee, and if additional hospitalization is needed after that, an additional lifetime reserve of 60 days can be used at a higher coinsurance payment.

In addition, if a resident spends the requisite three qualifying days in the hospital prior to nursing home admission, Medicare Part A will pay for up to 100 days of nursing home care. However, many individuals get confused on this point. First, there has to be, at a minimum, three inpatient hospital days during which the person was admitted to the hospital and was under treatment, not just observation. Furthermore, the person needs to meet qualifying standards in which he or she can no longer stay in the hospital yet has medical needs that cannot be met at home, and these must be documented by the attending physician.

Finally, Medicare Part A will pay for the first 20 days of a skilled nursing home stay in full and will pay for days 21–100 after an out-of-pocket copay expense on the part of the resident or family. The copayment for day 21 to 100 for 2012 was $144.50 per day for each benefit period and will increase to $148 in 2013 (Medicare.gov). The resident is not guaranteed 100 days of Medicare coverage, and the nursing home physician has to continuously certify that the resident continues to meet the higher level of care for Medicare coverage.

Medicare Part B is not automatic coverage, although older adults tend to select this coverage at a nominal monthly premium. Medicare Part B is supplemental coverage to Part A, and it helps to pay for some physician office visits, testing, home health services, and other medical services and equipment.

Although Medicare Part A usually generates greater revenue, Part B also plays an important role in nursing care facilities. During periods when the person may need certain occupational, physical, or speech therapy and may not be covered by Part A, Medicare Part B is an important supplement that can pick up the cost of these services. Caps have been introduced for Medicare Part B services, especially for occupational, physical therapy, and speech services. In 2012, the cap for occupational therapy was $1,880.00. Physical therapy and speech therapy are together, and, again, in 2012, the cap for combined services in this area was $1,880.00 (*www.cms.gov/Research-Statistics-Data-and-Systems/Statistics-Trends-and-Reports/NationalHealth ExpendData/index.html?redirect=/NationalHealthExpendData/25_NHE_Fact_Sheet.asp*).

In Medicare Part C, often referred to as Medicare Advantage, individuals sign up with a healthcare plan that also provides Medicare, often an HMO plan. In so doing, individuals may get some additional coverage that Medicare does not typically provide.

MEDICAID, MEDICARE, AND THIRD-PARTY PAYMENT

Medicare Part D, which went into effect January 1, 2006, offers prescription coverage to seniors. Although much of the plan was devised to support the noninstitutionalized population, Part D has had an effect on the long-term care industry. Starting January 1, 2006, those who were dually eligible, meaning that they had Medicare but were also receiving coverage under Medicaid, especially in relation to their long-term care pharmaceutical needs, now have their pharmaceutical costs paid under Medicare Part D.

Medicare Part D was developed as part of the Medicare Modernization Act, which attempted to address important deficiencies, especially pharmaceutical or prescription coverage, which failed to exist under Medicare. It is a market-driven plan that created prescription drug plans (PDP). Because Medicare Part D was set up to take advantage of competitive market forces to keep prices down, the PDPs will become prescription insurance plans for particular regions, developing their own formularies and setting their own monthly premiums. This new development will pose an important new, and probably complex, change to long-term care. At this time, it is too early to evaluate its effect.

Medicare reimbursement

As mentioned earlier, payment under Medicare has moved from a retrospective payment system to a prospective payment system, which is often referred to as PPS. The Balanced Budget Act of 1997 introduced a system of payment in which resident care was reimbursed on a daily basis with specific payment categories into which the resident was placed. The Minimum Data Set (MDS) system is important for determining Medicare reimbursement.

Residents were placed into resident utilization groups or RUG categories. The initial RUG system was a 44-group classification scheme with specific reimbursement rates for each of the 44 groups. This has currently expanded to 66 different RUG categories. This PPS is somewhat similar to the DRGs that were introduced in the early 1980s, and it created a system of reimbursement in nursing care facilities that is tied to the specific category in which a resident is placed. The location of the facility, based on city/metropolitan or rural area, as well the facility's geographic location within the country, also affects reimbursement rates for the same RUG level. In other words, two residents in the same RUG category would have the same level of reimbursement in the same city but may have different reimbursement levels depending on whether the facility is in a rural versus urban or suburban area or in the Midwest versus the Western part of the United States. Finally the RUG score that determines the level of reimbursement is generated by the assessment and MDS process.

A brief example will help to illustrate the RUG process. Let's say that Resident A lives in a nursing home in the same state as Resident B. But Resident A's nursing home is in a suburban area and Resident B's nursing facility is in a rural area. Both have a RUG score for the first 15 days of the month at rehab ultra high level (RUC) based on their clinical and rehabilitation status. This score carries a daily reimbursement of $442 for Resident A and $402 for Resident B. If both were reevaluated and both received a new RUG score of rehab high (RHC) to be calculated for the rest of the month, Resident A could receive a daily reimbursement from RHC of $332 and Resident B could receive a daily reimbursement rate of $301 due to their different geographic locations.

This example demonstrates two cases, each with the same clinical status and prospective payment grouping but different reimbursement based on the nursing facility's geographic location. Furthermore, the federal government and the Centers for Medicare & Medicaid Services (CMS) determine the specific rates attached to the RUG classifications as well as any differences due to geographic locations. We will discuss the PPS, consolidated billing, and the MDS process in more detail in a separate chapter.

Meeting Medicare requirements

Medicare Part A is an entitlement program, or a form of federal insurance for people who are at least 65 years of age. However, certain people with other disabilities, such as blindness or kidney disease, who are younger than 65 may qualify for Medicare Part A as well. Medicare Part B is an optional insurance program. Those who are eligible for Part A also become eligible for Part B. But where Part A provides automatic entitlement upon meeting certain requirement standards, Part B must be paid for by those who choose to take Part B. Medicare Part A pays for inpatient hospital care, skilled nursing facility (SNF) care, and hospice care. Medicare Part B covers a significant level of physician services, certain home healthcare, as well as certain diagnostic tests, such as laboratory tests and x-rays.

Medicare Part A, often called the hospital insurance portion of Medicare, differs in its level of coverage for hospitals, nursing facilities, and hospices. For example, hospital coverage can extend for 90 days, with the possibility of 60 lifetime reserve days that can be used. For nursing facilities, the coverage limit is 100 days; the first 20 days are paid in full, and days 21–100 have a copay attached to their use. As mentioned, in 2012 the copayment was $144.50 for days 21–100.

Medicare benefit periods

Medicare coverage is based on "benefit periods" during which residents are eligible to receive hospital and nursing home care (LTC-Resources.com). As mentioned, the benefit period for nursing home care covers a

MEDICAID, MEDICARE, AND THIRD-PARTY PAYMENT

possible 100 days. Another benefit period is not allotted to the resident until 60 days after the end of the prior benefit period. Furthermore, for a resident to be eligible for SNF care and Medicare reimbursement:

- The resident must be hospitalized prior to admission to a nursing facility for three consecutive days, not counting the day of discharge

- The resident must be admitted to a nursing facility within 30 days of his or her hospitalization

- The physician must certify the resident's need for skilled nursing care

- The resident must require a daily skilled service, such as physical therapy, occupational therapy, or speech therapy, and skilled nursing care outside of normal nursing care

Hospice care is also covered under Medicare Part A. It is covered under "periods of care," and residents qualify as long as a physician certifies that they are terminally ill and probably will have less than six months to live (LTC-Resources.com). The periods of care cover two 90-day periods, which in turn are followed by an unlimited number of 60-day periods, as long as the resident's physician continues to certify that the resident meets the criteria for being terminally ill. Therefore, for a resident to be continued on Medicare Part A for hospice services, the resident must be initially certified and recertified as necessary to continue receiving the Medicare benefit.

Clearing up a Medicare misconception

A common misconception that occurs when a resident is discharged from a hospital to a SNF is that the resident or his or her family thinks the resident is entitled to the full 100 days of Medicare reimbursement. First, as noted earlier, the first 20 days are covered in full, but days 21–100 have a copay attached to them. Second, although the person may be transferred from the hospital and may qualify for skilled coverage under Medicare Part A, he or she still has to meet stringent requirements to continue being covered under Medicare. The resident is evaluated on days five, 14, 30, 60, and 90, and during any one of these evaluations, if the multidisciplinary team feels the resident no longer requires skilled services, billing under Medicare must be discontinued.

To continue to maintain a person under Medicare when the person is not benefiting from skilled care on any level would be fraud. Thus, the facility's interdisciplinary team should meet regularly to protect against this egregious error.

CHAPTER 11

The administrator's role in the billing process

The healthcare administrator usually does not involve him or herself in the total Medicare billing process. Because it is so complex, administrators at most long-term care facilities have their accountants or professional billing personnel submit billing information to a CMS designated national repository. Nevertheless, administrators do have to be aware of a few major elements. First, the administrator should be somewhat familiar with the MDS process. Although a nurse is usually in charge of the MDS process, the administrator has to make sure MDS personnel are fully capturing everything that can be billed for and are not short-changing the facility because they are not capturing the true complexity of the resident evaluation process, possibly leading to a lower RUG score and, consequently, less revenue.

This means the evaluation process, through the use of the MDS, is a driving force for Medicare billing, and often it may not capture everything that could be coded for in the MDS process, leading to a potentially lower reimbursement level. This is not to say that the administrator should encourage MDS personnel to code for things that are nonexistent. However, the administrator should be able to help choose well-informed personnel to oversee this area, as well as to address, in an informed manner with MDS personnel, whether the facility is capturing the true RUGs.

The administrator also must be able to calculate revenue from Medicare, especially Medicare Part A. The administrator may be directly involved in this or may oversee someone else who handles this. Revenue for Medicare services is calculated at the end of the month. Often, before the revenue is sent to the accountant or billing personnel to be submitted to the national repository, the administrator or MDS personnel (or both) review the month's productivity, review the RUG levels and days of Medicare for the month, and calculate the appropriate RUG billing amount for the number of days associated with each RUG category. Physical or occupational therapy personnel also can play an active role in this process. This helps to provide for a greater level of internal control. After the MDS coordinator compiles this data, it is further reviewed by the administrator and possibly calculated by either the administrator or the MDS personnel and finally reviewed together before the information is sent to billing personnel.

One final element the administrator should understand has to do with the day-to-day rules the long-term care facility must incorporate into its internal accounting process. The administrator must remember that not everyone qualifies for the full 100 days of Medicare and must be able to explain this information to residents and family members. Furthermore, the administrator must understand the concept of Medicare technical denials. This happens when the resident has not had the appropriate number of qualifying

MEDICAID, MEDICARE, AND THIRD-PARTY PAYMENT

hospital days or the resident no longer qualifies for Medicare because he or she has exhausted his or her Medicare days in a relevant benefit period.

Demand billing

Along with the aforementioned rules, the administrator must also understand the concept of demand billing. Demand bills are submitted by nursing facilities to the fiscal intermediary (FI) on behalf of the resident when the resident or his or her responsible party feels the resident should still be covered under Medicare even though the facility has stated that the resident no longer qualifies for Medicare coverage. Although the resident still may have Medicare days available, the facility may terminate Medicare skilled care services because it feels the resident no longer meets the qualifications to remain on Medicare paid services.

Upon terminating the resident from Medicare services for reasons other than technical denials, the facility is obligated to inform the resident that he or she has the right to demand billing and contest the termination of Medicare with the FI. Upon waiting for the Medicare FI to render a determination, the facility is allowed to bill the resident only for the coinsurance or deductibles the resident may have to pay. The facility is not allowed to bill for the full amount of the services until the facility and resident are informed of the FI's final decision.

Demand bills differ from one facility to another and from one population of residents to another. Therefore, you should keep a monthly demand billing log, signed by you, MDS personnel, and the bookkeeper/admissions personnel, attesting to the demand billing issue for the month, as well as keep these individuals informed as to the demand billing on a current level. This is a simple procedure in which a form is devised and is completed at the end of each month. The form should include the total demand bills for the month, and it should have a place for a cumulative total for the year to date to be entered. This form also aids Medicare billing personnel, who are often contracted outside your facility and who want to be made aware of any demand billing for the month. In addition, it helps during survey time when surveyors want to see information on demand billing; keeping an organized, monthly record of demand billing helps to facilitate the survey process.

Reconciliation reports

CMS expects you to provide quarterly and annual reconciliation reports. You complete the quarterly report on a CMS 838 form, which reports any credit balances that may be owed to Medicare due to excess Medicare funds received. For example, say a hospital received payments for John Doe that totaled $5,000 more than what was appropriate. This $5,000 would have to be reported and repaid to CMS.

CHAPTER 11

Another example would be a nursing facility that receives Medicare funds for a resident who no longer qualifies for Medicare reimbursement. Both of these examples demonstrate a credit balance owed to Medicare that needs to be reported and eventually paid. In addition to the quarterly reconciliation, a larger annual reconciliation is required that is much more detailed and must be completed by someone who has a good deal of expertise in accounting.

The annual reconciliation addresses issues of cost accounting of the healthcare facility for the particular fiscal year. Medicare and RUG scores are also addressed in greater detail in the regulatory section due to their importance in long-term care.

Managed care billing

Many healthcare administrators as well as other healthcare professionals have been increasingly deluged by an array of managed care organizations. The rise in managed care has perhaps been the area of greatest change in the healthcare landscape in the United States. Given that our healthcare industry has typically been based on free-enterprise medicine and retrospective reimbursement, the increasing influence of managed care with the intention to manage the rising inflationary cost of healthcare has become a prevalent and prominent feature in our healthcare industry.

Today, slightly more than 14% of the U.S. Gross Domestic Product comes from the healthcare industry, with an annual per-capita expenditure of approximately $5,000 (Cockerham 2004). HMOs are the most common type of managed care organizations. Given this diverse third-party source of payment, the administrator has to be aware of the different managed care systems and possible reimbursement issues associated with them. Of course, it is impossible to be aware of every third-party payment source and their parameters for healthcare reimbursement, especially in long-term care. But the administrator has to make sure that the admissions staff checks out the levels of reimbursement and type of insurance providers that may exist before a resident is accepted.

Frequently, insurance companies may have to be contacted to see whether they are willing to reimburse a resident for your long-term care services. Sometimes insurance companies may ask whether you are willing to enter into a one-time resident contract, with weekly or bimonthly reevaluation and renewal. Again, you must weigh the costs and benefits of entering into such a situation. Admissions personnel will have to follow these cases closely with insurance caseworkers, and possibly after the insurance company denies any further claims, admissions personnel may have to assist with disenrollment, whereby the resident who still may be in need of long-term care has to be disenrolled or canceled out of his or her insurance plan to institute Medicaid enrollment for continued long-term care.

MEDICAID, MEDICARE, AND THIRD-PARTY PAYMENT

Third-Party Payment

Facilities can lose money that is owed to them by not assessing a resident's copayment. With Medicare, as well as with most insurance plans today, managing cost is an issue. Because of this, copayments are part of our healthcare environment.

When working through the monthly billing process, it is important to look for potential copayments that are due to your facility. If Medicare or a third-party payment source exists, immediately look to see whether a copay exists. When healthcare staff members see money coming into the facility, such as large Medicare checks or insurance reimbursements, they see the value of their work and a sense of elation and satisfaction results.

However, always look beyond the obvious, for additional copays could be due for services rendered that you have overlooked. In reality, if you and your bookkeeper are paying close attention to your accounts receivable and its related aging documents, this creates a process that sensitizes the bookkeeper toward developing a mind-set to continuously look beyond the obvious and look at what is often missing.

Look out for potential improprieties

A comment should be made regarding the need to guard against potential improprieties. The administrator has to monitor for dubious practices by physicians as well as other staff members. For example, the Stark Law, or Ethics in Patient Referrals Act of 1989, prohibits physicians from making patient referrals to other areas where the physician may have a financial interest. Say, for example, that a physician refers a patient to a lab that the physician owns or refers a hospitalized patient he or she has been taking care of to a nursing home he or she owns. Each of those referrals may be viewed as a violation of Stark Law.

Also, the administrator has to guard against potential kickbacks that have been found to exist in the healthcare industry. The anti-kickback statute is a federal law that penalizes those who engage in kickbacks. Basically, it states that people cannot solicit, induce, or simply give something for getting something in return, especially when Medicare and Medicaid funding is involved. For example, a physician makes an agreement with a local hospital that if it steers nursing home residents to his or her nursing facility, he or she will in return provide the hospital with frequent use of its laboratories for all the facility's Medicare residents; this type of quid pro quo relationship would violate federal law under the anti-kickback statue.

12 The Financial Implications for Insurance Policies

In addition to surety bonds, which we discussed earlier in this book, the healthcare administrator has to be aware of some other forms of insurance that are required to support the daily operation of a long-term care facility.

Property Insurance

Property insurance insures against physical damage to the building and the property on which the building resides. A property insurance policy assists with monetary reimbursements for damage due to fire, vandalism, wind, tornadoes, and other types of weather. At times, these policies are tailored to the geographic area in which the facility is located, as there may be some expected differences between policies for facilities located in certain areas of the United States. For example, hurricane coverage may be more explicitly addressed for facilities on the East Coast than for facilities in the Midwest, and vice versa for tornado insurance.

Because of the recent terrorist attacks that have transpired in the United States, many insurance companies are now addressing this in their policies. It is feasible that healthcare facilities, especially large hospitals, could be susceptible targets of such attacks. Therefore, many policies now include provisions of coverage for potential issues related to terrorist activities.

Liability Insurance

Liability insurance is an important form of insurance that administrators must understand fully. Liability insurance usually is in the form of general liability insurance and professional liability or malpractice insurance.

CHAPTER 12

General liability insurance covers claims that may be filed against your healthcare facility by workers, visitors, or other individuals who may become injured on the premises. For example, a visitor to your facility who slips and falls on ice, fracturing her pelvis, may sue the facility. In this case, general liability insurance helps to provide coverage.

Conversely, professional liability insurance provides coverage against patients or family members of patients who are filing suit, claiming that the facility was negligent in the provision of care that led to the injury, illness, or death of the patient. This insurance would be used when a family stated that the patient died from a surgical procedure that went awry or that the patient's bedsores are directly attributed to poor and negligent care on the part of the healthcare facility. Today, because malpractice litigation has become common, tort reform has been initiated in many states to prevent patients or families from suing for outrageous amounts of money.

Many insurance policies also will target special coverage areas, such as transportation and vehicle liability coverage. Many healthcare facilities use vehicles to transport patients to other facilities or even to activities. These plans separate themselves from the other insurance plans because now individuals are moving outside the facility. Therefore, many insurance companies will address these special forms of coverage under a separate plan.

Workers' Compensation

Workers' compensation is another insurance plan that is mandated by states. This type of insurance provides medical and financial coverage for workers who have been hurt while carrying out their job duties. It does not cover workers who hurt themselves outside their job. The amount of workers' compensation a facility pays is based on its history of worker injuries. It is important for the administrator to have some knowledge of the workers' compensation laws of the state in which the facility resides, as well as perhaps a copy of the workers' compensation law for ready access when needed.

Taxes

Taxes are important for most industrialized societies. Many of the programs the government provides, along with many subsidies, can be offered only because of the taxes collected from individuals and businesses. Businesses, especially partnerships, corporations, and limited liability companies, become acutely aware of this when they have to file with the IRS to obtain a federal employer identification number (EIN). This is the number that is used on all federal tax forms.

THE FINANCIAL IMPLICATIONS FOR INSURANCE POLICIES

The state in which your healthcare facility is located will also provide you with an EIN for filing your state taxes. Taxes are complex to understand, and this is why there are specialists in this area to assist you with your business' tax issues. However, as a healthcare administrator, you should have some basic knowledge of taxes, and, therefore, we will cover a few of the more prominent tax concepts related to healthcare administration.

Employers are responsible for matching the federal Social Security and Medicare taxes that are paid by their employees. Employers also must make contributions based on a percentage of their employees' wages to the Federal Unemployment Tax Act. The IRS will establish a tax payment schedule for your business. Through the use of Federal Tax Deposit Coupons Form 8109, you are required to submit regular payments to a specified bank, which then sends your tax payments to the federal government.

Businesses do not pay their taxes directly to the IRS but instead make arrangements with a bank to send their deposit coupons and checks for tax payments. The business—in this case, the healthcare facility—is obligated to submit a quarterly payroll tax return, known as Form 941, which reconciles its tax payments with the wages that were paid. Form 941 must be submitted each quarter in a timely manner. The IRS imposes severe penalties for being late in filing this form.

When employees start working, they fill out a W-4 form, which establishes their federal tax burden. They also fill out tax withholding forms for state taxation. At the end of the year, the business must furnish each employee with a W-2 form, which explains the amount the employee earned in wages as well as the amount he or she contributed to taxes. Federal law states that a W-2 must be submitted to each employee annually, and no later than January 31 of the new year. The W-2 for the total workforce in your facility also must be submitted to the Social Security Administration, along with form W-3, no later than February 28. Also, federal form 940, which deals with the reconciliation of unemployment taxes that were paid for the year, must be sent to the IRS annually.

Another tax form that is important to understand is the 1099 form. There are a few different types of 1099 forms, but for this section we are concerned with the miscellaneous or 1099 MISC form. If you hire an independent contractor who works outside your facility and is paid more than $600, or if your contractor is not a corporation, you must file a 1099 MISC form (Mose, Jackson & Davis 1997).

Contractors that have the distinction of being limited liability companies (LLC) are treated as partnerships and not as corporations, and therefore will need to have a 1099 MISC filed for the services they rendered.

CHAPTER 12

When you hire independent contractors, always have them fill out a W-9 form so that you have the name under which they are doing business as well as their tax identification number. This will aid in filling out the 1099 form. Each year, all 1099s must be sent to contractors no later than January 31 and to the IRS by February 28.

Just as individuals file tax returns, businesses file tax returns based on the category of business in which they have been classified for tax purposes. Most healthcare facilities are corporations. A corporation is established by the state in which the healthcare facility is located by filing articles of incorporation with the state. This creates the healthcare facility as a separate entity from those who work for the corporation. It becomes a legal entity in and of itself separate from those individuals who make it up. Incorporating is often the chosen method of establishing a business, because it minimizes liability to people who work for the corporation. Ownership is established through the sale of stock, and those who run the corporation are usually separated from those who own the corporation.

Contrary to the corporation, business entities that are sole proprietorships, owned by a single individual, or partnerships are less often found in the healthcare environment. Liability firmly rests with those that own the business enterprise. Because the healthcare environment is litigious, this could lead to a person who was a sole proprietor, or an individual who ran a healthcare facility based on a partnership, potentially losing all of his or her life's assets. Tax laws and forms that need to be filed are also different for proprietors and individuals than for corporations.

Some healthcare businesses are LLCs. These companies often share the limited liabilities of corporations yet have many properties of partnerships, including being treated similar to partnerships for taxation purposes. Another newer distinction similar to the LLC is the limited liability partnership (LLP), which licensed professional practices will use because they usually are not able to use the LLC distinction under many state tax laws. Many physicians may enter LLPs, which provide limited liability to partners. This arrangement prevents partners from also being liable due to another partner's negligent practices.

13 Consolidated Billing, the Prospective Payment System, and the MDS

With the Balanced Budget Act of 1997 (BBA) that was officially instituted in 1998, and with the Balanced Budget Refinement Act of 1999, a new era of billing came into place for long-term care facilities. Services under Medicare Part A now became part of a "bundled" case mix prospective payment system (PPS), and payment was based on a prospective payment for the category in which the resident was placed. Retrospective billing and "unbundling" services such that others could bill for services rendered to nursing home residents no longer was able to exist. Now the skilled nursing facility (SNF) had to bill for a resident's care under Part A. This eliminated a tremendous amount of duplicate billing that was previously a major problem when services were unbundled and being billed by other vendors who would provide the services. It essentially created a greater centralization for services and placed billing accountability in the hands of one unit, the SNF, which would be responsible for submitting the financial information to the fiscal intermediary. The consolidated billing process is far from an easy system to understand and work with, however. And although administrators need to understand the basic features of how the system works, in reality most facilities have professional billing personnel to take care of this information.

Consolidated Billing

As of October 1, 2010, the new version of the resident assessment instrument took effect. The new version, MDS 3.0, replaced MDS 2.0. The consolidated billing process is still driven by the Minimum Data Set (MDS). The number of resource utilization group (RUG) categories that the SNF bills for has expanded from 53 case mix categories to 66 in total. Furthermore, with MDS 3.0, the MDS data are no longer transmitted to the individual states but rather to a national repository.

Administrators need to understand a few basic rules when dealing with the consolidated billing system. The 7/5 rule states that residents must receive skilled nursing care seven days each week and rehabilitation

CHAPTER 13

services five days each week for Medicare Part A reimbursement under the skilled consolidated billing system. The midnight rule states that the facility is allowed to bill for all Medicare Part A residents who are in bed at midnight. The three-day qualifying stay says that a person who has Medicare Part A must have been admitted to a hospital for three qualifying days before he or she can be covered under Medicare Part A within a nursing home. If the person qualifies for admission, there is a 30-day rule for transferring him or her to a nursing facility from the hospital. If the person meets the three-day requirement, Medicare Part A coverage will continue to exist for admission to a skilled nursing home for 30 days from hospital discharge.

Once the person is admitted, Medicare Part A will pay for up to 100 days, following a 20/80 split, with the first 20 days covered in full and the last 80 days covered with a copayment that is needed. Confusion here results when many people feel they are guaranteed a full 100 days. No such guarantee exists, and they must meet criteria to remain on Medicare. For a person to be able to qualify for a full 100 days of Medicare Part A, they must follow the 60-day break of illness rule, which states that to requalify the person must not have skilled coverage in the nursing home or hospital; in other words, the person must be free from skilled intervention for a minimum of 60 days. These are just a few of the rules that exist, but these in particular are rules that the administrator should understand.

A skilled service that can be covered under Medicare Part A for skilled nursing home admission falls into at least one of three categories: overall management and evaluation, observation and assessment, or education and training. Overall management and evaluation is based on admission to a SNF where the physician care plan deems that it is necessary for the person to have skilled nursing services rendered and skilled rehabilitation services provided to aid the person in increasing his or her functional status.

A skilled service may be covered under the observation and assessment category when the individual needs to be observed, when there is potential for impending change, or when changes to the individual's treatment regime are imminent. A person can be skilled under education and training if he or she needs educational and training activities from nursing or rehabilitation to aid in enhancing his or her functional status. Remember that there must be interdisciplinary involvement in skilling residents for Medicare Part A reimbursement, and the care plans must be specific in addressing the goals for skilling a resident, as well as whether the resident is making progress toward achieving these goals. Failing to do so can lead to a loss of Medicare reimbursement.

CONSOLIDATED BILLING, THE PROSPECTIVE PAYMENT SYSTEM, AND THE MDS

It is important for administrators to have some working knowledge of services that are excluded from consolidated billing. These are services that are excluded from Medicare Part A bundling and often can be covered under Medicare Part B. The Centers for Medicare & Medicaid Services (CMS) has divided the exclusionary codes into five major categories:

- Category I: exclusion of services beyond the scope of a SNF

- Category II: additional services excluded when rendered to specific beneficiaries

- Category III: additional excluded services rendered by certified providers

- Category IV: additional excluded preventive and screening services

- Category V: Part B services included in SNF consolidated billing

Within the preceding categories are the following services that are excluded from Part A consolidated billing:

- Physician services furnished to a SNF resident

- Services provided by physician assistants

- Services provided by nurse-midwives

- Certified nurse anesthetist services

- Psychiatric and qualified psychological services

- Institutional dialysis services and supplies associated with these services within the SNF setting

- Epoetin alfa and darbepoetin alfa (drugs used for end-stage renal disease)

- Hospice care within a SNF

- Preventive services (can be billed to Part B)

- Outpatient hospital emergency room services

CHAPTER 13

- Ambulance trips that transport for SNF admission or to home, as well as to select outpatient procedures

- Designated hospital outpatient procedures that are often billed by these agencies

- Chemotherapy and administration services

- Radioisotope services

- Customized prosthetic devices

Remember that although these services are excluded from consolidated billing under the Part A PPS, some of the services can be billed under Part B services if appropriate under specific guidelines, such as certain preventive services. Also, some services can be captured under Medicare Part A, but they cannot be provided within the SNF, such as hospice. Furthermore, other services may also be billed separately by the vendor that services the resident off the SNF campus, but it is not part of the consolidated billing protocol for the SNF.

As you can see, most individuals who are involved in billing are specialists, and the healthcare administrator needs to be in close contact with these individuals. Although administrators do not have to be experts in the specific revenue codes that are used or commit to memory the various codes that are used on the billing forms, they should be somewhat aware of why they are needed. The administrator should be aware of what the health insurance prospective payment system (HIPPS) code is, as this becomes the basis for knowing what the Medicare Part A revenue is for the month. HIPPS consists of a three-letter RUG code and a two-letter assessment code. The first three letters are important, because they can tell you at a glance where the resident stands on his or her RUG levels. They provide a quick understanding of the skilled level of care that is being given within the SNF and potential reimbursement for the month.

MDS Drives All Billing

The MDS drives not only consolidated bill but also all billing. The MDS is a federal OBRA requirement that must be performed on all residents, regardless of whether they are skilled under Part A. Therefore, although administrators do not have to be experts on MDS, they must have a basic understanding and be conversant on MDS as well as hire people who are qualified to carry out the MDS and who understand the importance of MDS coding.

CONSOLIDATED BILLING, THE PROSPECTIVE PAYMENT SYSTEM, AND THE MDS

The MDS process is a very intricate coding process that needs professionals who are meticulous and who code with the utmost scrutiny. All residents must have an MDS completed on them regularly. Those who come into a facility and are not being skilled by Medicare must still have an initial comprehensive survey that is completed on them no later than 14 days, with care plans completed no later than seven days after the initial comprehensive MDS. After the initial MDS, a resident must have a quarterly MDS assessment, not to exceed 92 days, and each year the resident must have a comprehensive MDS assessment not to exceed 366 days from the last annual assessment.

When a person comes in and is skilled under Medicare Part A, the schedule is different. There must be a five- and 14-day MDS assessment, followed by a 30-, 60-, and 90-day MDS assessment if the person continues to utilize Medicare. Nurses must complete daily Medicare charting, with an emphasis on the skilled issue; MDS coding should strongly reflect the skilled issue as well. The MDS assessment does not have to be completed exactly on the five-, 14-, 30-, 60-, and 90-day schedule, and the regulations do give some parameters for each assessment. Figure 10.1 depicts a typical Part A assessment schedule.

Assessment Type	Assessment Reference Date	Billing/Reim. Period Covered
5-Day Assessment	Days 1–5	Sets Payment Rate for Days 1–14
14-Day Assessment	Days 11–14	Sets Payment Rate for Days 15–30
30-Day Assessment	Days 21–29	Sets Payment Rate for Days 31–60
60-Day Assessment	Days 50–59	Sets Payment Rate for Days 61–90
90-Day Assessment	Days 80–89	Sets Payment Rate for Days 91–100

It is important to have a skilled MDS person who can set correct assessment reference dates (ARD), which become the common point of reference for look-back periods, which can be five, seven, 14, or 30 days. Many areas of the MDS assessment will ask you questions regarding the resident's condition over the previous seven, 14, or 30 days from the ARD. For example, Section D, which looks at mood and whether the resident is depressed, has a look-back period of two weeks from the ARD.

Also, on five-day MDS assessments, the reference period can extend back during the hospital stay and needs to be counted. Many make the mistake of counting only the nursing home days. This can result in a big reimbursement loss. For example, if the resident was being treated with IV therapy in the hospital and was part of a 14-day look-back period, the person needs to count back from the ARD even if it includes hospital days. Because of the skilled nursing and rehabilitation that the resident received during this

CHAPTER 13

period, this could place the resident in a higher reimbursement category. Furthermore, it is not correctly capturing the information that is requested for that look-back period. Many individuals on the interdisciplinary team are responsible for filling out the MDS assessment, and this makes it critical to have an MDS person who checks each MDS for accuracy when it is completed.

Off-Cycle Assessments

Off-cycle assessments come in many flavors. One off-cycle assessment is the Other Medicare-Required Assessment (OMRA). OMRAs are performed on residents who can no longer be skilled under a rehabilitation category, yet they have significant nursing issues that Medicare Part A will continue to cover. Many individuals refer to this as skilling the resident under nursing. If the person can still be covered under Medicare Part A for skilled nursing services when they can no longer be covered under rehabilitation, the OMRA must be performed one to three days after the discontinuation of rehabilitation services. A new ARD is set on either the eighth, ninth, or tenth day after the discontinuation of rehabilitation for the OMRA.

Two other off-cycle assessments are the Significant Change in Status Assessment (SCSA) and the Significant Correction of Prior Assessment (SCPA). An SCSA is done when there is a significant decline or improvement in the resident's status. Typically, significant changes in status impact two or more areas in a resident's overall health status. Upon discovering that a significant change has taken place, an SCSA must be completed within 14 days. The SCPA is used when a significant MDS error has been discovered in the coding process on either a full or a quarterly assessment. The SCPA is really a correction of an assessment to make it reflect the true condition of the resident and make sure adequate data submission is completed to the state agency. Furthermore, adequate coding needs to be reflected so that proper reimbursement can be obtained.

Administrator Involvement

As mentioned earlier, MDS assessments are an important and mandatory element of the nursing home process. Administrators should make sure they are involved, in collaboration with billing and MDS personnel, in examining at least weekly whether the assessments have been sent to the respective repository, whether there are any issues, and whether the billing and MDS information matches. An MDS must be submitted to the national repository no later than 14 days after its completion. It is important that the administrator understands that a nurse must be the MDS personnel. Although a licensed practical nurse can be an

CONSOLIDATED BILLING, THE PROSPECTIVE PAYMENT SYSTEM, AND THE MDS

MDS coordinator or MDS nurse, only an RN can sign the completed MDS and certify it. This is why most facilities often defer to having the full-time MDS personnel or director being an RN. So, in addition to having an individual who is knowledgeable in MDS and coding, it often is very beneficial to have an RN head the MDS area since an RN is ultimately responsible for signing and attesting to MDS correctness.

A Maze of RUGs and Minutes

The current MDS RUG IV comprises 66 individual RUG codes. The major RUG groups fall into eight categories and have been changed from MDS 2.0. These eight major categories are as follows: Rehabilitation plus extensive, Rehabilitation, Extensive services, Special care—High, Special care—Low, Clinically complex, Behavioral symptoms, Cognitive performance, and Reduced physical function.

FIGURE 13.1
MDS RUG-IV GROUPS AND SOME OF THE COMMON ASSOCIATED CODES

RUG Group	Codes	Features
Rehab Plus Extensive	RUX, RUL, RVX, RVL, RHX, RHL, RMX, RML, RLX	Rehabilitation such as PT, OT, SP, and extensive services.
Rehab	RUC, RUB, RUA, RVC, RVB, RVA, RHC, RHB, RHA, RMC, RMB, RMA, RLB, RLA	Rehabilitation such as PT, OT, and speech.
Extensive Services	ES3, 3ES2, ES1	Tracheostomy and ventilator/respirator use; Tracheostomy or ventilator/respirator use; isolation for active and infectious diseases.
Special Care—High	HE2, HD2, HC2, HB2, HE1, HD1, HC1, HB1	Comatose and completely ADL dependent; septicemia, quadriplegia, parenteral/IV fluids.
Special Care—Low	LE2, LD2, LC2, LB2, LE1, LD1, LC1, LB1	Multiple sclerosis with ADL scores of > than 5; Parkinson's disease with ADL score > 5; feeding tube.
Clinically Complex	CE2, CE1, CD2, CD1, CC2, CC1, CB2, CB1, CA2, CA1	With or without depression and varying levels of ADL scores.
Behavioral Symptoms and Cognitive Performance	BB2, BB1 BA2, BA1	Cognitive impairment found in BIMS score of less than or equal to 9 or on the Cognitive Performance Scale (CPS) of greater than or equal to 3. Or evidence of hallucinations and delusions. Or physical or verbal behavioral symptoms toward others, other behavioral symptoms, rejection of care or wandering.
Reduced Physical Function	PE2, PE1, PD2, PD1, PC2, PC1, PB2, PB1, PA2, PA1	Restorative nursing services for urinary and/or bowel training; passive/active range of motion (ROM); amputation/prosthesis care/training; splint or brace assistance; dressing and grooming training; eating and swallowing training.

CHAPTER 13

It is very important that information is coded properly. The RUG grouper software establishes the RUG level after the data have been entered. For the rehabilitation groups, the first two letters indicate the type of rehabilitation level: RU stands for Rehab Ultra High, RV stands for Rehab Very High, RH stands for Rehab High, RM stands for Rehab Medium, and RL stands for Rehab Low. Also, a specific number of rehabilitation minutes needs to be met to qualify for the particular levels as well as therapy five times per week. To meet the RU category, a person must have a minimum of 720 minutes of rehab per week; for the RV category, a minimum of 500 minutes per week; for the RH category, a minimum of 325 minutes per week; for the RM category, a minimum of 150 minutes per week; and for the RL category, a minimum of 45 minutes per week. In addition, there are also activities of daily living (ADL) scores that are associated with each RUG level, but due to the extensive nature, it is not included in this book. However, this is another change under MDS 3.0. With MDS 2.0, there were 18 ADL levels. With the new version, MDS 3.0, 16 ADL levels exist.

The Importance of Certification

Individuals are not guaranteed Medicare A coverage. As mentioned, qualification requirements must be met, such as a three-day hospital stay, placement within a nursing home within 30 days of the three-day stay, and having a therapeutic intervention that is needed for rehabilitation and skilled nursing care. It is important here to have an initial physician certification, which is the physician's documentation that indicates the necessity for such care. As mentioned, the person must receive five days of rehabilitation and/or seven days of skilled nursing care to be eligible.

For a resident to continue to receive Medicare Part A coverage, they also must continue to qualify for Medicare coverage. After the initial certification, the first recertification must be completed no later than 14 days after admission by the attending physician. Afterward, there is a 30-day rule that states further recertification must be completed no later than each 30-day period from the previous certification. Certification, recertification, rehabilitation, and nursing documentation needs to specifically address the rehabilitative and skilled nursing care plans in terms of why the person continues to need these services. Also, skilled rehabilitation and nursing services have to demonstrate the efficacy of the treatment to justify continued Medicare coverage. Failure to do so is another reason claims may be denied.

CONSOLIDATED BILLING, THE PROSPECTIVE PAYMENT SYSTEM, AND THE MDS

The New Version—MDS 3.0

As previously mentioned, starting in October 2010, MDS 2.0 was phased out and MDS 3.0 was phased in. The goal of MDS 3.0 was to provide an evaluation tool that allows for more interaction in the evaluation process. There was a shift from relying more on residents' records for evaluations, which was more common with MDS 2.0, and a movement to more standardized interviewing of residents with MDS 3.0. The goal continues to be the same: to have a comprehensive tool that is part of each resident evaluation.

MDS 3.0 has employed some new terminology that is different from MDS 2.0. The formerly known Resident Assessment Protocol (RAP) is no longer part of 3.0. The new terminology is Care Area Assessment (CAA). There are 20 CAAs in version 3.0. The Care Area Trigger (CAT) alerts the evaluator of the need to conduct further assessments in particular areas through use of the CAAs.

As mentioned, MDS 3.0 is built on greater resident participation in the evaluation process. Also, attempting to devise an instrument with greater accuracy based on the resident's own personal comments is very important. Attempting to standardize how the interview process with the resident is done was of major importance, and, therefore, this led to many new standardized interviews. Some of the major new changes that have taken place in this area are as follows:

- Section C, dealing with cognitive patterns, now relies on an instrument built in to MDS 3.0, called the Brief Interview for Mental Status (BIMS). This attempts to standardize the use of a single instrument to evaluate each resident's cognitive status.

- Section D addresses mood using a standardized mood interview built into the MDS process, referred to as the PHQ-9. This relies on the assessor asking the resident a standard and invariant set of questions that do not deviate from one resident assessment to another.

- Section F is referred to as Preferences for Customary Routine and Activities. Again, this section has been added and uses a standardized interview format to obtain the resident's response on issues of importance related to having snacks in between meals, choosing their own clothes to wear, whether listening to music is important, or whether being able to keep up with the news is important, just to name a few items.

- Section J deals with pain assessment, and it uses a standardized interview with the resident built in to the MDS. When the resident is able to provide verbal information in this area, he or she is asked

CHAPTER 13

standardized questions dealing with pain presence, pain frequency, pain effect on function, and pain intensity. Since pain is a subjective experience, the goal here is, when the resident is able to provide answers, develop a pain program based on his or her subjective experience from the information received through the interview data obtained from the resident.

- In section Q, a brief interview is based on evaluating the resident's wishes about returning to the community. If he or she is able to provide answers to questions, MDS 3.0 requests that the interviewer ask, "Do you want to talk to someone about the possibility of returning to the community?" This is part of the section that deals with Participation in Assessment and Goal Setting, consistent with providing the resident with greater self-determination over his or her therapeutic plan of care.

The minimum data set or MDS 3.0 is a very comprehensive tool that has been developed to provide thorough evaluations of residents. MDS 3.0 requires that the interviewers provide greater weight to the specific questions that are asked of the residents. The MDS instrument has always been a comprehensive tool, and it remains as such. To end this section, I want to provide the reader with a brief overview of the sections that MDS 3.0 covers. They are as follows:

- Section A is identifying information, such as race, ethnicity, age, language spoken, marital status, type of assessment, etc.

- Section B deals with assessing hearing, speech, and vision.

- Section C addresses cognitive patterns and, as mentioned earlier, is one of the sections that uses the standardized interview, in this case the BIMS.

- Section D examines mood and makes use of the standardized interview using the PHQ-9 to evaluate the resident's mood.

- Section E deals with behavior and examines whether hallucinations or delusions are present; whether physical, verbal, or violent behavior exists; whether they are amenable toward care; as well as whether wandering occurs.

- Section F examines preferences for customary routine and activities. Here again, the standardized interview is used to provide information on preferences that the individuals has for their lives within the nursing home environment.

CONSOLIDATED BILLING, THE PROSPECTIVE PAYMENT SYSTEM, AND THE MDS

- Section G deals with activities of daily living. This looks at many important behaviors, such as walking, eating, bed mobility, toilet use, and dressing and how much if any assistance or supervision is needed for the resident in conducting these tasks.

- Section H examines bowel and bladder habits of the resident. Are they continent or incontinent for stool or urine? How often does this problem exist? And do they use devices such as a catheter?

- Section I addresses the active diagnoses that the resident has over the past seven days.

- Section J is referred to as health conditions. An important area in this section is conducting the standardized pain interview on the resident. It also assesses for tobacco use, prognosis, and fall history.

- Section K addresses issues of swallowing and nutritional status. It documents height, weight, and whether weight loss exists. It documents signs and symptoms of swallowing issues that may exist, use of special diets, and oral and dental status.

- Section M looks at skin conditions. It evaluates the pressure ulcer risk of the resident, whether any pressure ulcers exist and at what stage, and the integrity of one's skin.

- Section N is concerned with the type and administration of medications that the resident receives.

- Section O examines special treatments, procedures, and programs that the resident uses. For example, it examines chemotherapy and radiation, oxygen therapy, BiPAP and CPAP usage, transfusions, and dialysis, to name a few. This is also an important area that examines physical, occupational, and speech therapy needs, respiratory needs, and restorative nursing programs that are used on the resident.

- Section P deals with use of physical restraints on the resident, the type that is used, and the frequency of usage.

- Section Q examines the extent the resident was able to participate in the assessment, their discharge plans, and whether they have plans about returning to the community.

- Section V is the CAA summary area. It documents data from the most recent prior OBRA assessment. It also requests which one of the 20 CAAs was triggered and whether it was addressed and care planned.

CHAPTER 13

- Section X is referred to as the correction request area.

- Section Z is called Assessment Administration, and it documents the HIPPS and RUG version code as it relates to pertinent billing information. It also requests that all persons involved in completing the assessment sign and date it with their sections completed. Finally, it requests an RN signature, usually the MDS coordinator, to sign and date the form, verifying assessment completion.

14 Quantitative Analysis for Long-Term Care Administrators

Quantitative analysis examines data through mathematical or numerical computation. Quantitative analysis uses various statistical and mathematical procedures to help analyze operational situations that administrators and managers encounter. It is very important for healthcare administrators to have some working knowledge of some important forms of quantitative analysis.

The second half of this book will examine some important quantitative procedures to help the long-term care administrator analyze data more efficiently and effectively. It also provides the administrative professional with important scientific management skills, skills that have created management as a science—based on scientific skills—for making sound management decisions. This chapter is an introduction to some of the basic concepts of what science is, which may help to illuminate why management is a science devoted to making informed decisions rather than relying on intuition. The chapters that follow examine specific quantitative skills that are far from exhaustive but will provide the administrator with some basic quantitative skills that they can learn and master to help guide their decision-making within the healthcare environment.

Traditional Scientific Tenets

Before we examine some important concepts in quantitative data analysis, you should understand the basic principles of science. Again, modern management theory is based on science. Whether you are doing research in your organization, or whether you are in need of making decisions based on employing sound quantitative principles formulated on science, having a basic understanding of what the basic principles of science are will make you a more knowledgeable and competent administrator.

CHAPTER 14

Empirical evidence

Science is predicated on *empirical evidence,* or information we can verify with our senses. Empiricism is the cornerstone of all scientific investigation. For something to lend itself to scientific investigation, it must be observable and testable—thus, empirical. For example, demonstrating the efficacy of a treatment for decubitus ulcers often depends on measuring the ulcerated area to see whether any reduction has occurred, as well as noticing the integrity of the wound for such signs as granulation and epithelialization. All this is considered observable and empirical.

Objectivity

Objectivity is another important component in conducting scientific research. *Objectivity* is a state of personal neutrality when conducting research. When someone is objective, he or she does not impute any bias into the research or data analysis but rather examines the facts as they present themselves. Many times, especially in long-term care settings, nursing home and survey staff members encounter a level of disputation regarding this principle. Each is often guided by trying to observe the healthcare facility as he or she thinks it should exist, leading both groups away from objectivity and, consequently, toward the imputation of their own subjective biases.

Scientific determinism

The ultimate aim of scientific analysis is explanation. Thus, much of scientific investigation is based on trying to determine cause and effect. This is frequently called *scientific determinism.* Determinism is the position that relates every event to a preexisting set of events. It is a commitment to determinism that compels scientists to look for postulated mechanisms in the world. This commitment to determinism encourages scientists to define cause-and-effect relationships that are as inclusive as possible. The ultimate goal of science is to obtain an explanation for why something happened—what element (the cause) brought about the manifestation that is being studied (the effect). Most individuals who engage in scientific investigation, including healthcare administrators, will not always find the cause for a specific phenomenon, yet their obligation still rests on trying to determine that cause.

In many cases, the ultimate cause cannot, and will not, be found, and the best you can settle for is a correlation. Yet, you must always keep in mind that seeking an explanation for why a phenomenon occurred is the ultimate goal of scientific management.

QUANTITATIVE ANALYSIS FOR LONG-TERM CARE ADMINISTRATORS

The scientist usually gathers his or her facts via testing and retesting the phenomenon being studied. Scientists usually conduct several tests to gain additional confirmation of their results. This is because scientists must always maintain a reasonable amount of skepticism.

It is difficult and sometimes impossible to say that a theory has been proven beyond a doubt. Healthcare administrators and medical researchers deal with this by constantly retesting a hypothesis. If the test keeps coming back with the same results, support continues to be gained in favor of the hypothesis or theory that is being tested. This is how scientists gain a sense of assurance.

It's important to note that science is not a haphazard process, disconnected and random in its methods. It is focused, concise, and structured. At times, the systematization can be tedious, yet the tedious nature of science protects against random errors. Thus, science is based on step-by-step procedures that must be adhered to.

Parsimony

Parsimony is an essential principle that guides science. Parsimony means that, whenever possible, you should keep your scientific explanations as simple as possible. In other words, you should try to make your hypotheses, constructs, and operational definitions concise. Concept testing works best when the concepts are neat and compact and do not contain any unnecessary wordiness, which would make it difficult for the researcher (or healthcare administrator) to operationalize, or put the concepts into a workable frame, therefore making it difficult for those who are examining the research. Explanations also should be as exact as possible, avoiding any unnecessary hyperbole that will add to confusion.

In many ways, parsimony was influenced by the nominalist philosopher, William of Ockham. Ockham argued that when trying to explain the nature of something, one should not be more complex than necessary. In other words, we should avoid using more concepts than we need to explain a phenomenon. Ockham believed that the simplest explanation is most likely the correct one, although this is definitely not always true. This view came to be known as "Ockham's razor."

Ockham's razor helped to focus individuals and philosophers on looking at the observable and avoiding unnecessary and excessive use of words, ideas, concepts, and classifications that can complicate an explanation and thus confuse the understanding of the facts under consideration. Ockham's razor was an important concept that helped to create a path for more sophisticated scientific tenets to follow. One can see how parsimony was strongly influenced by Ockham's razor. However, it should also be mentioned that when research is being conducted on human behavior, it lends itself to a complicated nature that is often difficult to state parsimoniously.

Falsifiability

Before we discuss theory and hypothesis, we should discuss the scientific tenet of *falsifiability*. Karl Popper (1959), an Austrian philosopher, advocated the need for this scientific tenet. Since then, the concept of falsifiability has become a major principle that guides all scientific research. Falsifiability states that we can never prove that general statements or theories are true; however, we can prove their falsehood.

Most people believe that a good theory is one that can always be proven true, but this is a false premise. A theory that fails to lend itself to the concept of falsifiability is neither scientific nor a theory. A sound theory needs to be predicated upon the concept of falsifiability, because if the theory is wrong in any way, these falsehoods need to be found. This is important, because it helps to advance scientific explanation by eliminating those false explanations. Thus, we can say that a good theory is one that lends itself to being proven false if there is any problem with the theory.

Research Examined

Most scientific research deals with theories and hypotheses. A *theory* is usually a larger, general, and much more global explanation of something. It frequently is composed of many *hypotheses*, which are explicit statements regarding the expected relationships among variables. *Concepts* are abstract elements representing phenomena within the field of study. A concept is a packet of knowledge that holds an extensive meaning. Administration is often theoretically based, and theory is a driving force for determining how administrators will administrate and often evaluate their healthcare environment.

Usually a theory is too large and too general to test, so scientific investigation generally employs hypotheses. A good hypothesis details how one will measure the concepts that are under examination. A facility administrator, for example, may hypothesize that increasing behavioral intervention training for all of the facility's employees will reduce behavioral issues among patients in the facility, as found on the facility's quality indicator reports. By instituting behavioral intervention training and comparing quality indicator reports thereafter with baseline quality indicator reports prior to the introduction of training, the administrator can determine whether the behavioral intervention training was effective.

QUANTITATIVE ANALYSIS FOR LONG-TERM CARE ADMINISTRATORS

One major difference between the social, behavioral, and management sciences and the physical and biological sciences is that laws are frequently not part of the former. The physical and biological sciences frequently speak about laws, which are truly universal generalizations about classes of facts (Babbie 1998). However, laws in the social, behavioral, and management sciences are much more difficult to find, and when dealing with human and organizational behavior in a managerial context, they are almost impossible to find. Although laws are often elusive, all scientific investigation, whether physical or managerial, deals with facts. Sometimes facts and laws are confused. A fact is the objective, observable phenomenon that all scientific investigators work with. All sciences deal with facts as part of the observational unit of analysis, but as noted earlier, some sciences lend themselves more toward the development of laws than others.

Classifying research

Research can be classified by its type and purpose. The type and purpose of research can fall under four major headings:

- Exploration

- Description

- Explanation

- Prediction

Exploratory research

Exploratory research explores a particular topic. Often, especially when a researcher is trying to get a feel for a topic on which he or she may not have much information, exploratory research is used. This research is often used as a precursor to more extensive research or to examine whether it is worthwhile to engage in a research project in greater depth. Although many managerial researchers and healthcare professionals will use this exploratory research, it is less common for in-house administrative purposes.

Descriptive research

Descriptive research is used to describe situations and events. It helps to give individuals a better understanding of particular situations in which they may be interested. Descriptive research helps to describe characteristics of the population that are of interest to particular research projects and is more likely to be employed by healthcare administrators. For example, administrators may conduct a statistical analysis of the number and type of clientele using their emergency services over a six-month period, or they may conduct correlation research of their facility compared to other facilities and how staffing related to the number of citations received among the respective nursing facilities.

Explanatory research

Explanatory research tries to find reasons why certain things happened and is designed to provide causative explanations. Most healthcare administrators do not use explanatory research because of time constraints as well as possible ethical issues that may arise.

Predictive research

Predictive research tries to explain what will happen in the future if certain variables are manipulated. One of the major goals of science is to predict future events from known data. For the most part, administrators will use certain techniques to predict future events. For example, they may use regression analysis to statistically and econometrically forecast potential financial costs or future services that may be utilized at a given level.

As you can see, healthcare research can be conducted in many ways. These techniques are an important means of gathering data in the healthcare environment.

15 Common Quantitative Analytical Techniques for Healthcare Administration

Quantitative methodology is based on the application of numbers to analyze data. Through mathematical and statistical models and equations, healthcare administrators can obtain a significant level of information to aid in making important decisions. Many mathematical and statistical techniques are sophisticated and involved, and an in-depth discussion of them is beyond the scope of this book. Nevertheless, it is important for healthcare administrators to have a basic understanding of some of the more commonly employed quantitative techniques they will use.

Quantitative Methods

Three common quantitative methods that are used to describe data are the mean, median, and mode.

The mean

The *mean* is what most people think of when they think of an average. It is the sum of a set of scores divided by the total number of observations. For example, say you want to determine the average monthly census for the first five months of the year. If the first five months had a census of 90%, 75%, 83%, 92%, and 88%, you would add these scores and divide by five. As such, the mean score related to this batch of average census data would be 85.6%.

The following formula represents the mean:

$$\bar{X} = \frac{\Sigma X}{N}$$

Finance, Budgeting & Quantitative Analysis: A Primer for Nursing Home Administrators

CHAPTER 15

This formula is read Bar X, which represents the mean, and is equal to the summation of X divided by N. X represents all of the scores that have been summed (e.g., 90, 75, 83, 92, 88, which equals 428). This sum is divided by N, which represents the number of observations (e.g., five months, as used in the example above). Thus, 428 is divided by five, which is 85.6%.

The median

The *median* is just as easy to figure out. It is the score that is at the middlemost part of a distribution of scores—that is, 50% of the scores fall above the median and 50% fall below. For example, using the preceding example of census scores, you would find the median by first ranking the scores from highest to lowest—that is, 92%, 90%, 88%, 83%, and 75% (alternatively, you can rank them from lowest to highest). Given these scores, the median or middlemost number in the distribution is 88%.

Now, say you are examining the median census for the first six months of the year, resulting in the following monthly census data: 95%, 92%, 90%, 88%, 83%, and 75%. Remember that the median is the middlemost score in the distribution, where 50% of the scores fall above and 50% fall below. In this case, the middle would be somewhere between the third and fourth scores of 90% and 88%. Therefore, you would add these two scores and divide by two:

$$90 + 88 = 178 / 2 = 89\%$$

The mode

The *mode* is the score that appears most frequently in a given distribution. Say that for a given year the monthly census averages were as follows: 98%, 88%, 92%, 90%, 88%, 86%, 90%, 88%, 80%, 87%, 88%, and 90%.

In examining these scores, it is apparent that 88% appears four times, 90% appears three times, and all the other scores appear once. The mode for this distribution is 88%, because it is the number that appears with the greatest frequency.

Now say your monthly census averages for the year were as follows: 95%, 92%, 92%, 95%, 90%, 90%, 86%, 88%, 92%, 85%, 87%, and 90%. What number appears with the greatest frequency? Both 92% and 90% appear three times each, which is greater in frequency than 95% appearing twice and 88%, 87%, 86%, and 85%, all appearing once. Now two scores are appearing with the same frequency. The two

COMMON QUANTITATIVE ANALYTICAL TECHNIQUES FOR HEALTHCARE ADMINISTRATION

highest scores would demonstrate a bimodal distribution; therefore, the yearly census demonstrates two modal scores, 92% and 90%.

Visual Methods of Examining Data

Another way to examine data is to examine its distribution, or how it appears visually.

Summarizing data visually is common in scientific studies. Visual data leave a prominent impression in a person's mind. As such, administrators can often obtain important information for making decisions by examining data visually. In this section, we will discuss a variety of methods for examining data visually.

Skewness

Skewness measures the symmetry of a distribution. A perfectly skewed distribution of scores resembles a bell-shaped curve with the skew equal to zero. When the distribution of scores has a mean larger than the median, and when most of the distribution is loaded to the left, this is called a *positively skewed distribution*, and the skew is appreciably greater than zero. When a distribution of scores is loaded heavily to the right of the distribution and the mean is smaller than the median, this is a *negatively skewed distribution*, and the distribution is appreciably less than zero. Both positively and negatively skewed distributions are asymmetrical distributions.

It is important to examine the skew of a distribution, because it can tell you how data are distributed. For example, say you want to know how your facility compares to other facilities in the county in terms of number of citations received during the most recent census. Documenting the frequency of citations reveals that the citations fall into one of three patterns of skewness.

The following three diagrams demonstrate these three patterns. The x on the horizontal axis is where your nursing home exists in relation to other nursing facilities for citations received. As you move from left to right on the horizontal axis, a greater number of average citations are found.

CHAPTER 15

The following diagram shows that the nursing home is under both the mean and the median levels of average citations. This would be good news for you.

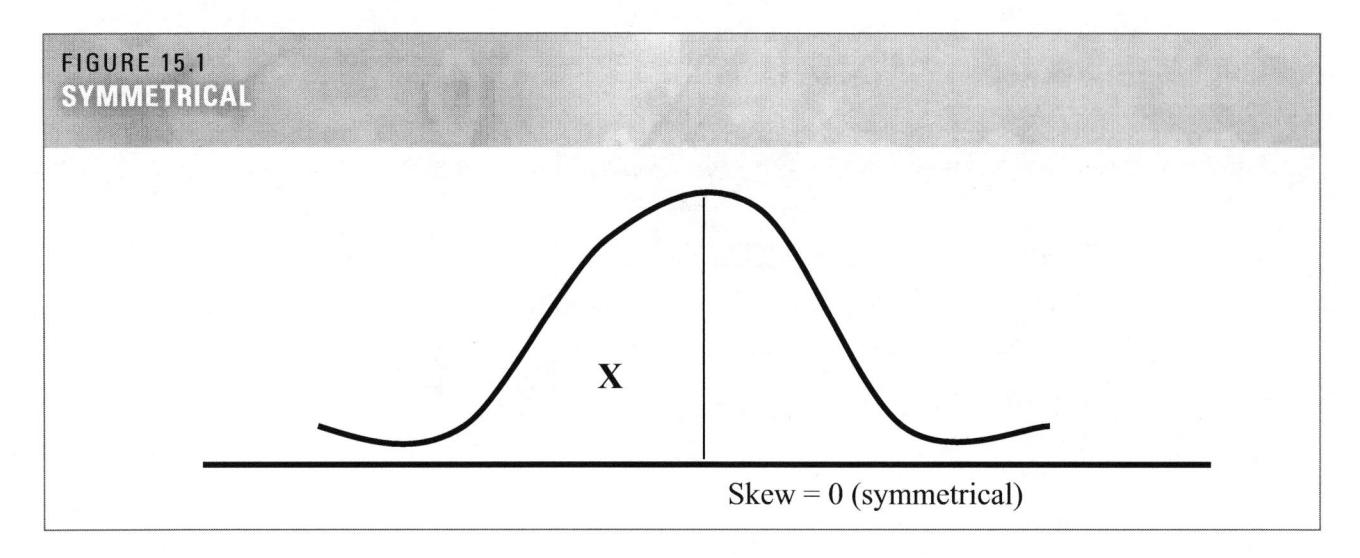

FIGURE 15.1
SYMMETRICAL

Skew = 0 (symmetrical)

You also can determine the skewness of a distribution by examining the direction of the tail in the distribution. In a positively skewed distribution, the tail runs to the right.

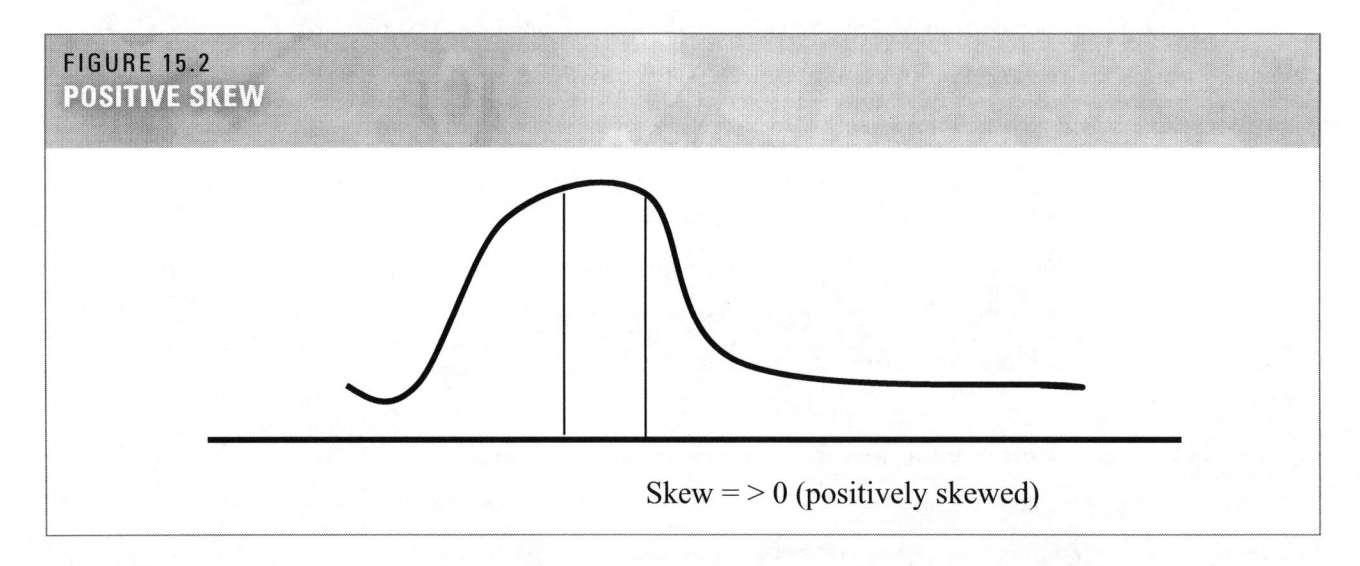

FIGURE 15.2
POSITIVE SKEW

Skew = > 0 (positively skewed)

Conversely, in the negatively skewed distribution, the tail runs to the left. In a symmetrical distribution, the scores are much more evenly dispersed throughout the distribution.

COMMON QUANTITATIVE ANALYTICAL TECHNIQUES FOR HEALTHCARE ADMINISTRATION

FIGURE 15.3
NEGATIVE SKEW

Skew = < 0 (negatively skewed)

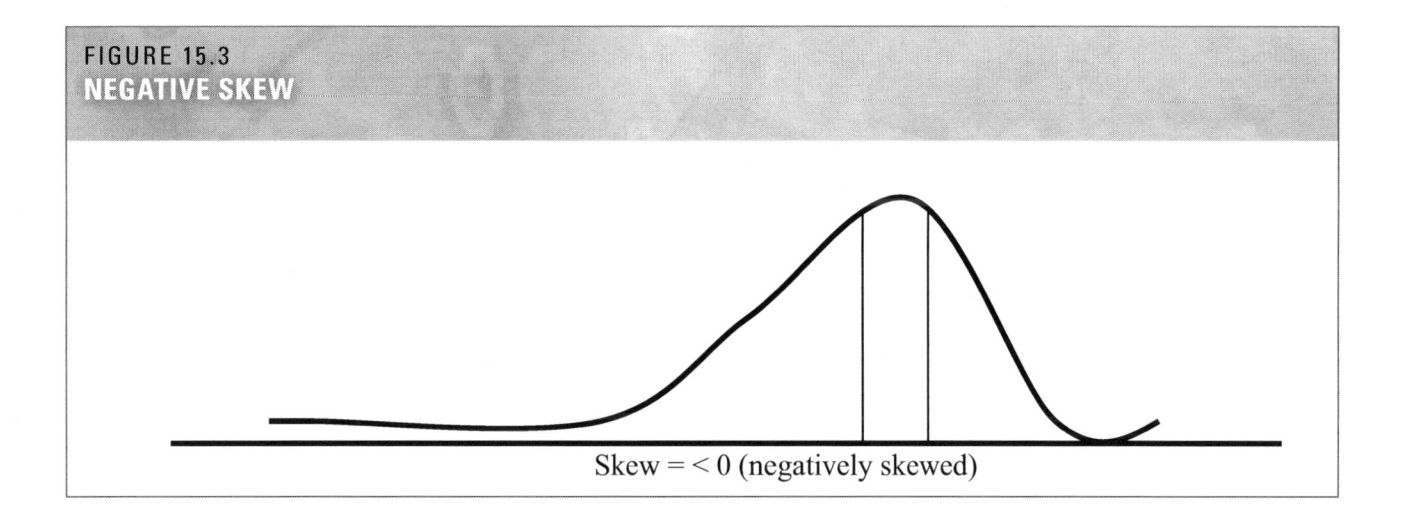

Kurtosis

Kurtosis also gives a visual depiction of a distribution of scores. However, kurtosis examines how peaked the distribution is in relation to the data being examined. For example, a normal bell-shaped distribution does not demonstrate a considerable amount of peak or flatness, and its distribution is often called *mesokurtic,* with kurtosis values close to zero. However, some distributions demonstrate a considerable amount of peak, where most of the scores are found within a small range of the center of the distribution. These distributions are called leptokurtic, and they have a kurtosis score that is considerably greater than zero. Finally, some distributions are flatter than normal distribution curves, and these are called *platykurtic*, with a kurtosis considerably less than zero.

To demonstrate, let's use the example that we used for skewness. Say you are interested in how your facility compares to others in the same county. In examining the data, you find that 25 of the 30 nursing homes in the area had little difference in the number of citations received, averaging approximately 8.9 citations. The other five nursing facilities were either much lower or much higher in number of citations received. Which type of distribution do you think would exemplify the results of this study? The distribution would probably look similar to the kurtotic diagram that demonstrates a greater level of leptokurtosis. The following diagrams demonstrate these three forms of kurtosis.

CHAPTER 15

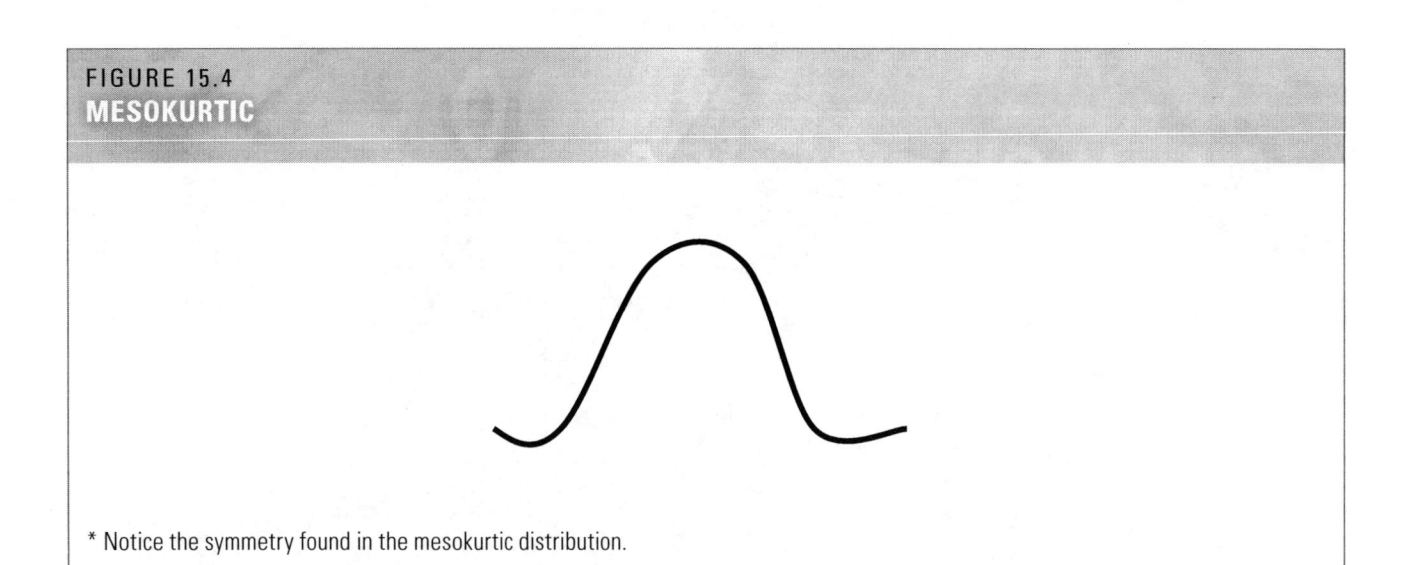

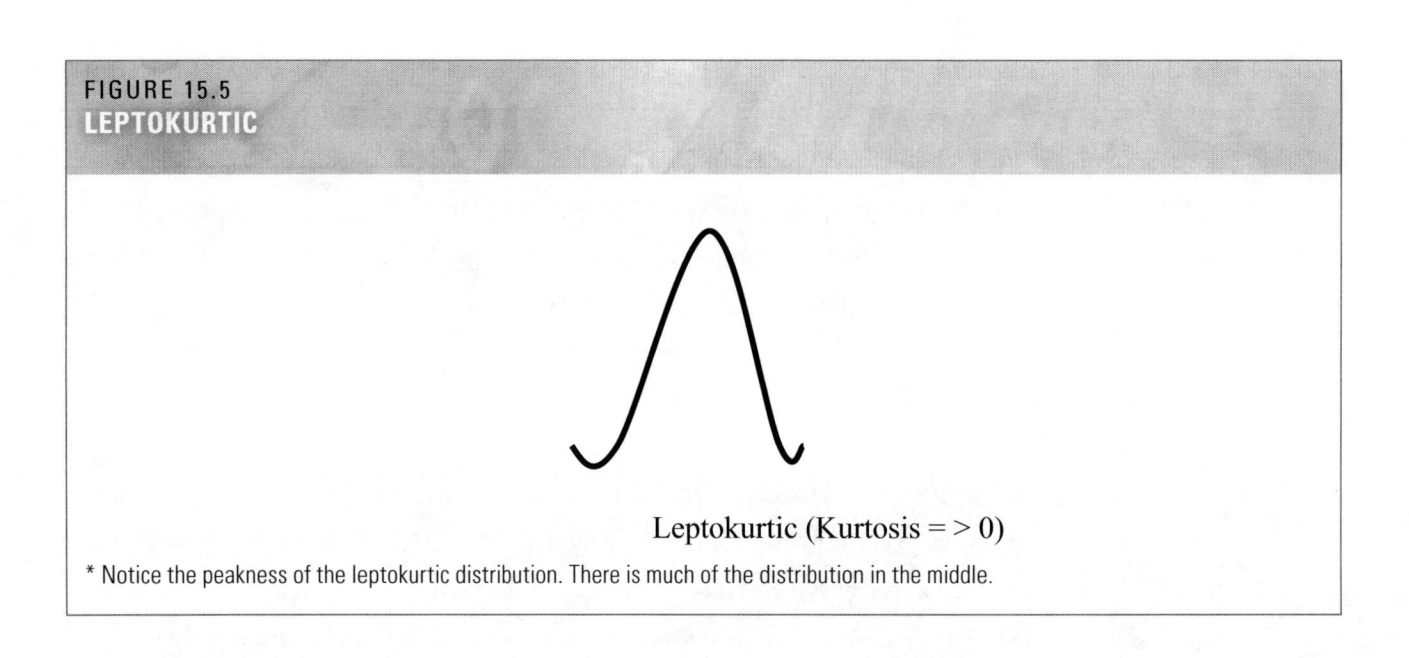

FIGURE 15.4
MESOKURTIC

* Notice the symmetry found in the mesokurtic distribution.

FIGURE 15.5
LEPTOKURTIC

Leptokurtic (Kurtosis = > 0)

* Notice the peakness of the leptokurtic distribution. There is much of the distribution in the middle.

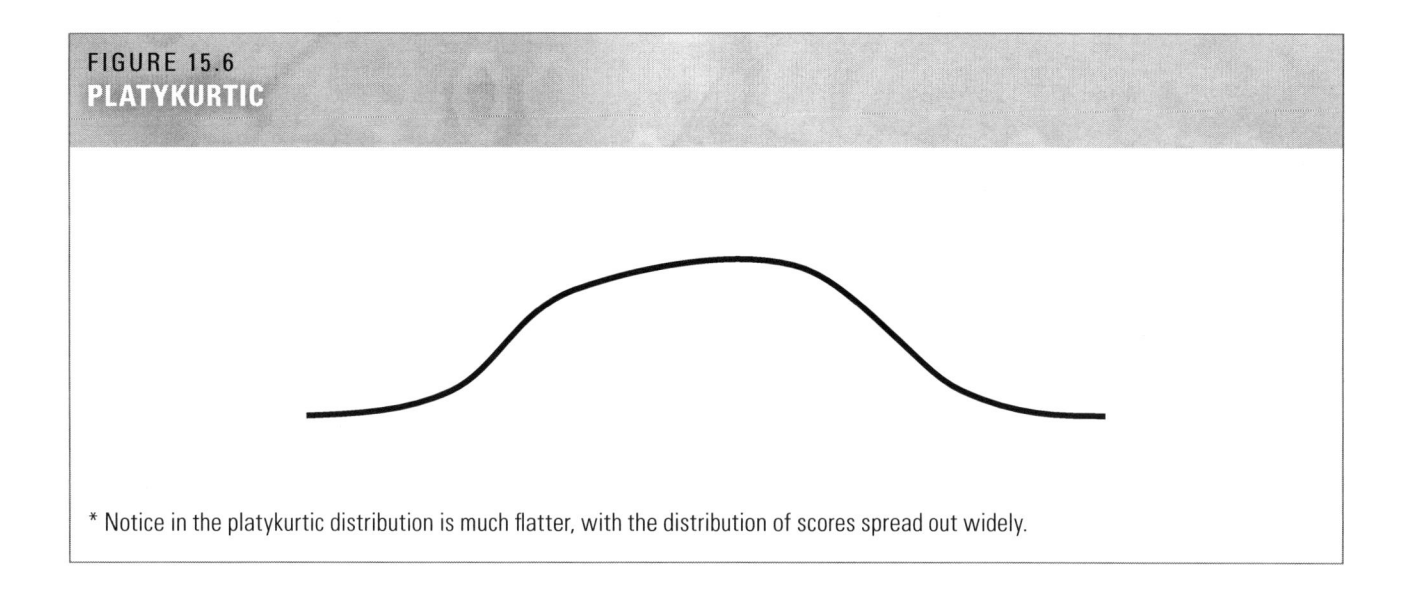

COMMON QUANTITATIVE ANALYTICAL TECHNIQUES FOR HEALTHCARE ADMINISTRATION

FIGURE 15.6
PLATYKURTIC

* Notice in the platykurtic distribution is much flatter, with the distribution of scores spread out widely.

Stem and leaf graphs

Stem and leaf graphs give the healthcare administrator an easy way to summarize data. They get their name through the analogy of how leaves grow out of the stems of plants. In this case, you would use a particular data interval as the stem, and a second digit of the numerical data as the leaf.

For example, say you and your director of nursing are examining the results of tests given to 20 nurses in your facility, dealing with baseline knowledge of psychotropic medication and its uses, classifications, and potential adverse effects to evaluate whether greater levels of training need to be instituted for the nursing staff. The scores for the nurses ranged from 50% to 98%. To simplify the data, you construct a stem and leaf graph. The following diagram demonstrates how to do this.

FIGURE 15.7
STEM AND LEAF GRAPH

STEM	LEAF
5	0, 2, 5
6	4, 5, 8, 9
7	0, 0, 5, 5, 5, 9
8	2, 5, 7, 7
9	0, 5, 8

CHAPTER 15

In the preceding diagram, the first row deals with the 50% range, with one nurse scoring 50%, a second scoring 52%, and a third scoring 55%. In the second row, one nurse each scored 64%, 65%, 68%, and 69%. In the third row, two nurses scored 70%, three scored 75%, and one scored 79%. Among those who scored in the 80% range, one nurse scored 82%, a second 85%, and two 87%. Finally, in the last row, one nurse scored 90%, a second 95%, and the final nurse scored the highest grade of 98% to lead the class.

As you can see, stem and leaf graphs help to simplify data by reducing it to a manageable level. Although it is not a highly sophisticated technique, it can help healthcare administrators organize their data into a clearer and more understandable framework.

Line graphs

A *line graph* or a *frequency polygon* is another good visual tool for data presentation. This type of graph looks at a particular variable and visually presents the frequency or number of individuals found in each category being measured.

Let's say you are interested in examining the frequency of incidents, on a month-by-month basis, that are found within your facility for a given year. You would like to engage in some descriptive research to summarize the incidents over the year. You could create a frequency polygon to represent the nominal frequencies found in the respective months, as shown in the following diagram:

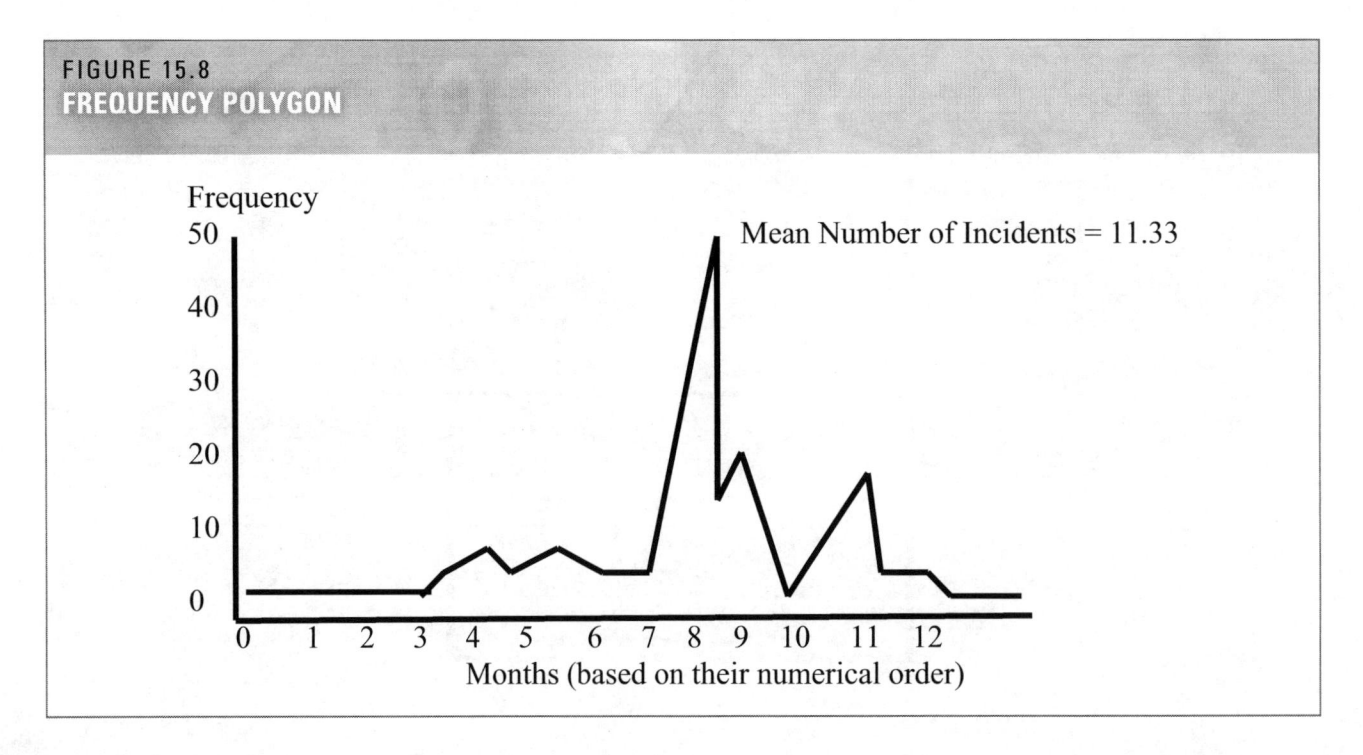

**FIGURE 15.8
FREQUENCY POLYGON**

COMMON QUANTITATIVE ANALYTICAL TECHNIQUES FOR HEALTHCARE ADMINISTRATION

Histogram

The *histogram* is another commonly used analytical tool to help give a visual display of data. Similar to a bar graph, the histogram is connected and continuous. Although it is a simple analytical tool, it can be helpful in conveying information visually. In fact, because it helps to visually enhance a person's explanation of data as well as being easy for others to understand, it is one of the most commonly used methods researchers use to present information.

The histogram can also be an important tool for healthcare administrators to assist them in providing a solid visual presentation of data. The following diagram demonstrates a histogram. It presents information similar to that found in the preceding frequency polygon. It is examining the number of resident incidents that happened during each month within a given year within a hospital. The only difference is now it is being visualized through the use of a histogram.

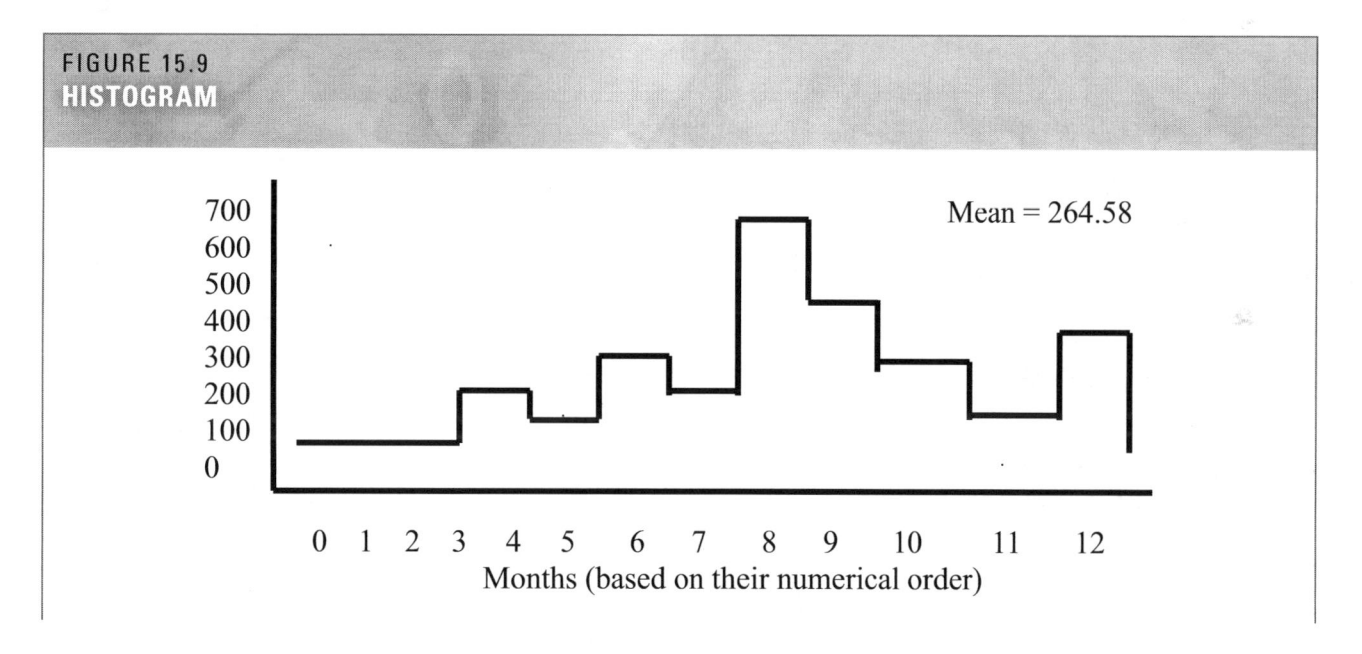

FIGURE 15.9
HISTOGRAM

Mean = 264.58

Months (based on their numerical order)

Examining Dispersion: The Spread of Scores

As you can see, when analyzing data, scores often demonstrate a considerable *level of variance or spread*. However, administrators may want to determine how dispersed the scores are and whether they are homogeneous or close together. One simple way to determine the spread of scores is through the use of a range. The range is equal to the highest score minus the lowest score.

CHAPTER 15

Say that over a six-month period you are interested in getting together with the director of nursing and examining your facility's monthly medication errors. The number of errors for each month is as follows: 5, 14, 10, 3, 8, 2. To determine the range, you'd place the numbers into an array, from highest to lowest: that is, 14, 10, 8, 5, 3, 2. Then you would subtract 2 (the lowest number) from 14 (the highest number), and you'd get 12, which is the range of errors over the six-month period being examined.

Standard Deviation

A more sophisticated way to examine data is through the use of *standard deviation*, which measures the spread of scores around a mean. Here is the formula for determining standard deviation:

$$SD = \sqrt{\frac{\Sigma(X - M)^2}{N}}$$

This formula reads as follows: The standard deviation is equal to the square root of the summation of X (the variable under consideration) minus M (the mean) squared, divided by N (the number of observations).

The standard deviation takes the individual scores and provides insight into the average deviation (spread) from the mean. Using the preceding example dealing with medication errors, the mean or average number of errors would be 7 for a six-month period. When you calculate the standard deviation using the preceding formula, you can see that the standard deviation is equal to 4.16, which for a small number of scores appears to be a fairly large amount of spread or dispersion.

To see how this would change, suppose that medication errors were examined again for six months and the following was found as a month-by-month average: 8.5, 5.8, 7.1, 4.5, 9.1, and 6.5. Notice that the spread of scores is considerably less, with a range of 4.60. The mean is 6.92, and with the lower dispersion or spread of scores, the standard deviation is reduced to 3.82. The following is a step-by-step procedure for figuring out the standard deviation. While reviewing these steps, remember that the mean is 6.92.

COMMON QUANTITATIVE ANALYTICAL TECHNIQUES FOR HEALTHCARE ADMINISTRATION

Step one: subtract the mean from each score as stated in the equation X – M.

X		M		
8.5	–	6.92	=	1.58
5.8	–	6.92	=	–1.12
7.1	–	6.92	=	0.18
4.5	–	6.92	=	–2.42
9.1	–	6.92	=	2.18
6.5	–	6.92	=	–0.42

Step two: Square each of the deviations as stated in the formula $(X-M)^2$

$(1.58)^2$ = 2.50
$(-1.12)^2$ = 1.25
$(0.18)^2$ = 0.03
$(-2.42)^2$ = 5.86
$(2.18)^2$ = 4.75
$(-0.42)^2$ = 0.18
                 ─────
                 14.57

Step three: The square root of 14.57, which is the sum of the square deviations:
$\sqrt{14.57}$ = 3.82

What does this spread of scores mean? To understand the greater significance of standard deviation, let's examine the following normal distribution, which is symmetrical and mesokurtic.

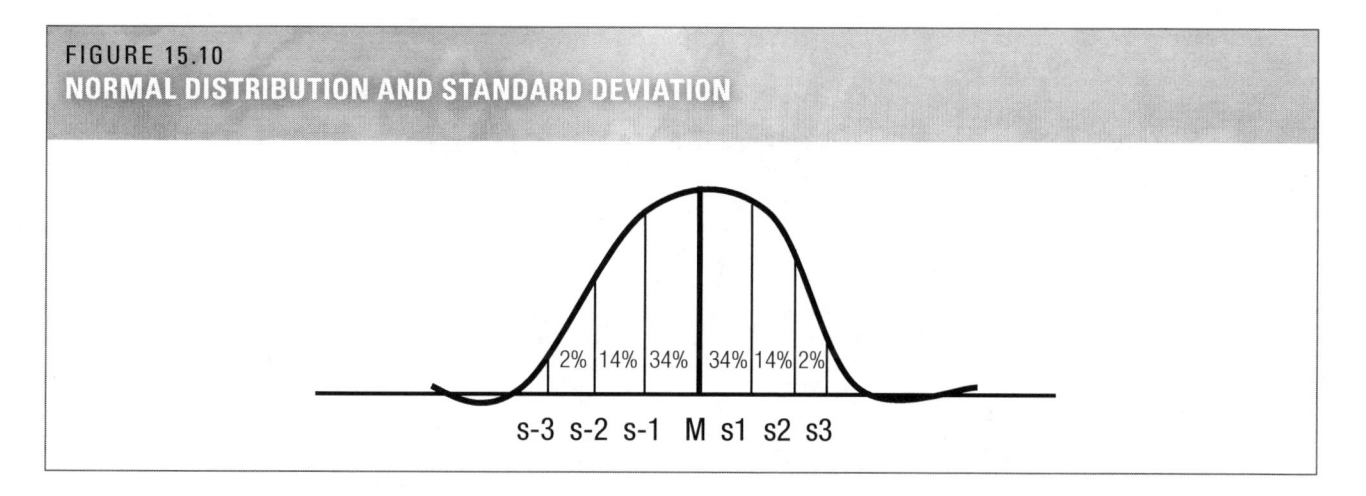

FIGURE 15.10
NORMAL DISTRIBUTION AND STANDARD DEVIATION

2% | 14% | 34% | 34% | 14% | 2%
s-3 s-2 s-1 M s1 s2 s3

In the preceding distribution, the middle area is represented by the average, or mean, scores. To the right, each line represents a standard deviation from the mean. All the scores on this side fall above the mean.

CHAPTER 15

On the left side, each line also represents a standard deviation away from the mean. Scores on this side of the distribution fall below the mean. Now notice the numbers inside the curve. These represent percentages that have been rounded off for convenience. On both sides of the mean, ranging from +1 to −1 standard deviation, the percentage of scores that fall below the mean and one standard deviation is 34%, and the percentage of scores that fall above the mean and one standard deviation is also 34%. Those that fall between +1 and −1 standard deviation units to +2 and −2 standard deviation units are 14%, respectively, on both sides. And finally, those scores outside of 2 standard deviations to 3 standard deviations on either side of the distribution account for about 4%, making up 2% roughly on each side of the distribution.

What does this all mean? Well, if you know the score is +1 standard deviation, you know the mean represents 50% of the distribution and that from the mean to +1 standard deviation unit is approximately another 34%. In other words, if you took a test and scored +1 standard deviation, you would have done better than 84% of the others who took the test.

Let's go back to our earlier example of medication errors. Our standard deviation was 3.82, and our mean was 6.92. Each standard deviation unit, either to the left or to the right of the mean, equals 3.82. Therefore, because the mean equals 6.92, one standard deviation above the mean equals 10.74, and two standard deviations above the mean equal 14.56. Conversely, one standard deviation below the mean equals 3.10. However, remember that the standard deviation gives us a rough average on the spread of scores as compiled from a number of scores. With that in mind, how would you compare a specific score to these results?

Well, you would now have to take each score, use the standard distribution you calculated, and convert it into a Z-score. The formula for the Z-score is as follows:

$$Z = \frac{X - M}{SD}$$

This formula reads that the Z-score is equal to X (which is the score we are evaluating) minus the mean (M), divided by the standard deviation (SD).

In this formula, X represents the score you want to examine, minus M, which is the mean, divided by the standard deviation. Using this formula, if we were to look at the May average of 9.1 medication errors, the Z-score would be equal to 9.1 minus 6.92, divided by 3.82, which equals 0.57 standard deviations above

COMMON QUANTITATIVE ANALYTICAL TECHNIQUES FOR HEALTHCARE ADMINISTRATION

the mean. Conversely, examining the month of April, where medication errors were below the mean, averaging 4.5, the Z-score would be calculated as such: 4.5 minus 6.92, divided by 3.82, which would equal −0.63 standard deviation units below the mean.

Using Z-scores helps to put a score into perspective regarding a larger distribution. Furthermore, because both scores in the preceding examples were the high and low scores and neither exceeded +1 or −1 standard deviation, you can see that the scores are packed tightly around the mean, with not a great deal of spread in the scores.

16 Correlation: The Importance of Measuring Relationships Between Variables

A common statistic that is often mentioned when measuring levels and strengths of association between two or more variables is *correlation*. I will not emphasize the mathematics behind correlation, although I will say that computing correlation is a laborious endeavor, usually due to the large amount of data the researcher is working with. However, computing even smaller amounts of data can be laborious as well.

Healthcare administrators can use correlation measurements by way of statistical formulas in their spreadsheet programs. Regardless of how you opt to compute correlation, however, it is important that you understand what it is and how it can be applied. In addition, although you can measure correlation in several ways, in this chapter we will focus on the most common method, the Pearson Product Moment Correlation Coefficient, developed by statistician Karl Pearson.

The Pearson Product Moment Correlation Coefficient

Before we get into the details of the Pearson Product Moment Correlation Coefficient, a bit of background information is in order. You measure correlation on a bipolar continuum, with a perfect negative correlation being –1.00 and a perfect positive correlation being +1.00. Zero correlation means no association exists between the two variables being examined. Also, a correlation cannot extend beyond –1.00 and +1.00. In addition, a positive correlation is not necessarily better than a negative correlation. As we will see, the positive or negative correlation deals only with how the two variables work in relationship to one another.

Finally, you should note that a perfect positive or negative correlation is rare; most correlations between variables fall somewhere between these two poles. These correlations are demonstrated in the following scatterplots, which are labeled as Figures 16.1, 16.2, and 16.3.

CHAPTER 16

FIGURE 16.1
PERFECT POSITIVE CORRELATION

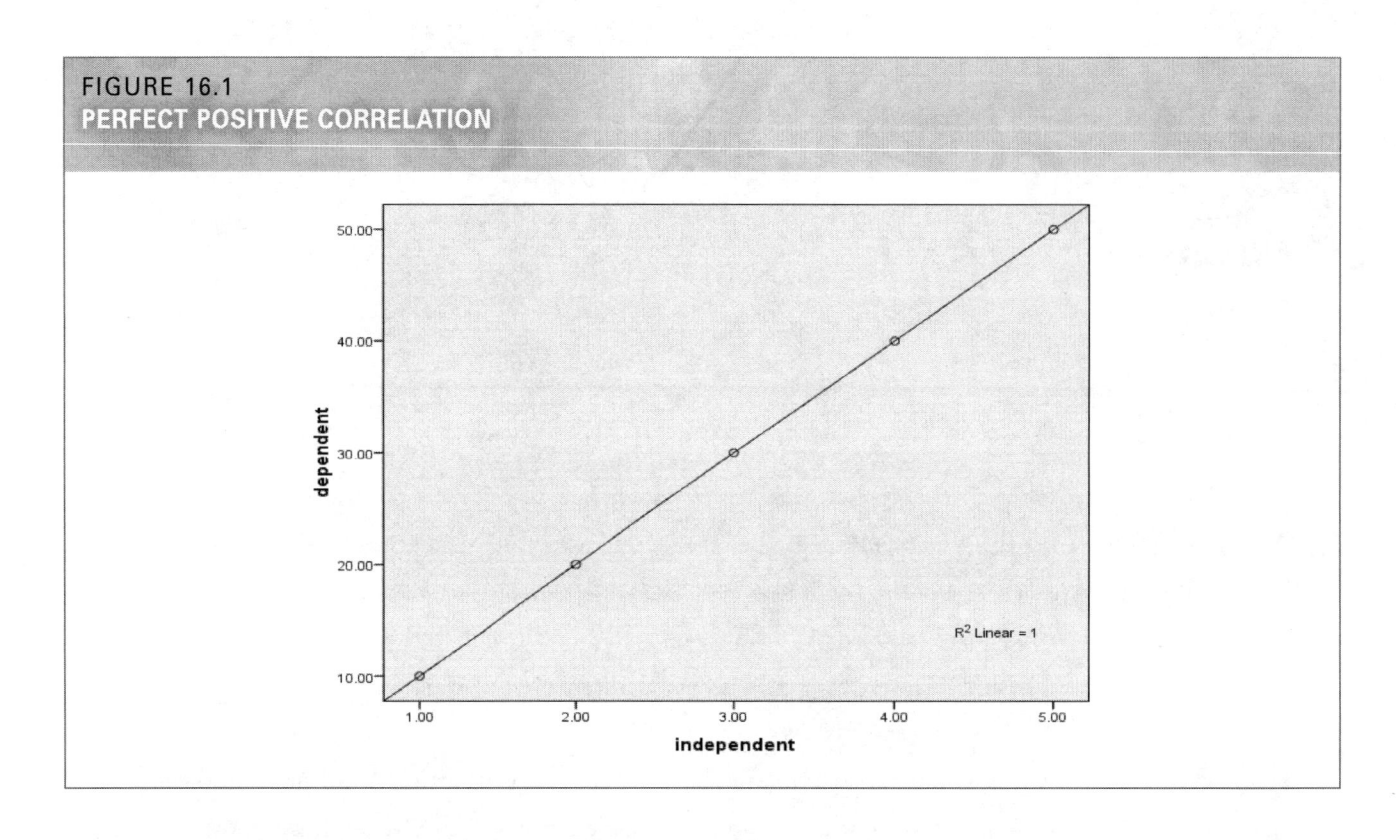

FIGURE 16.2
PERFECT NEGATIVE CORRELATION

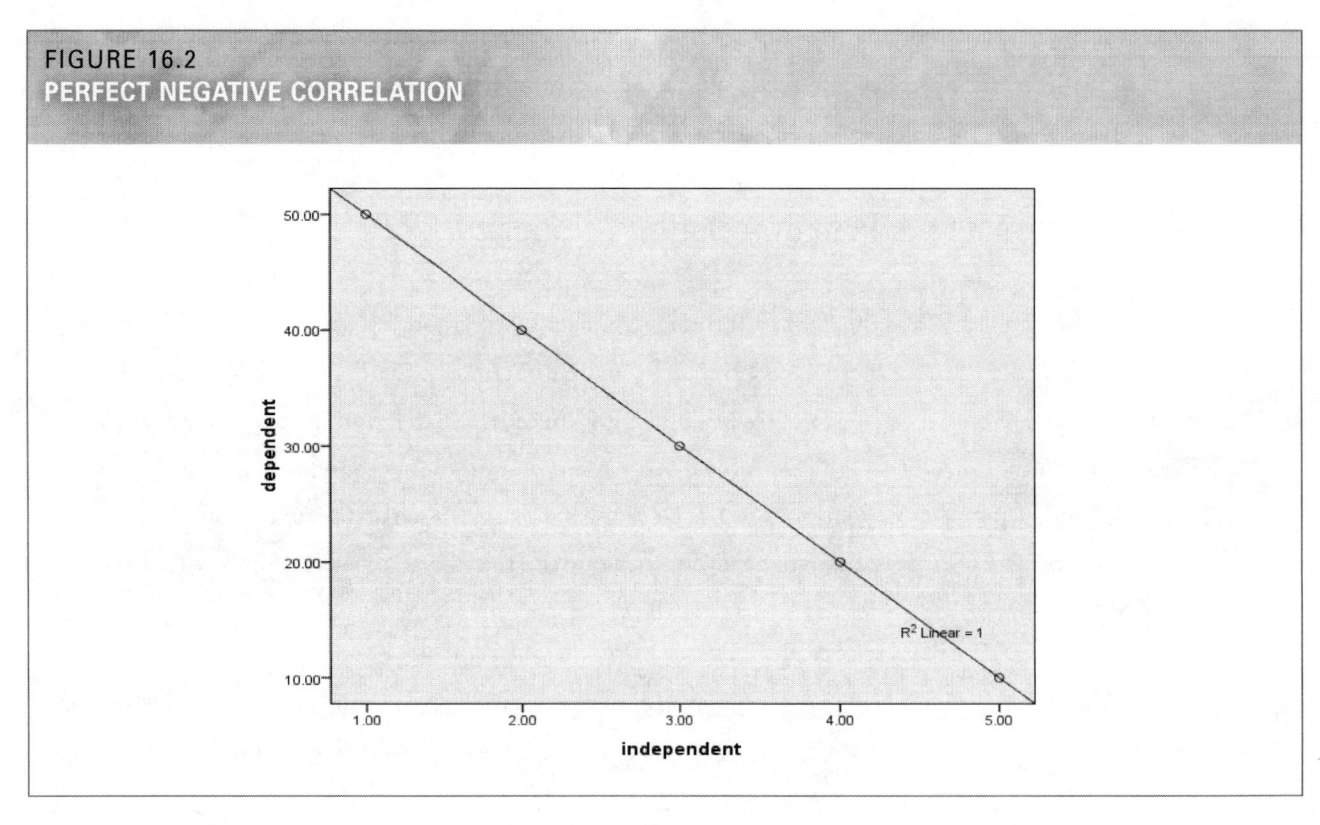

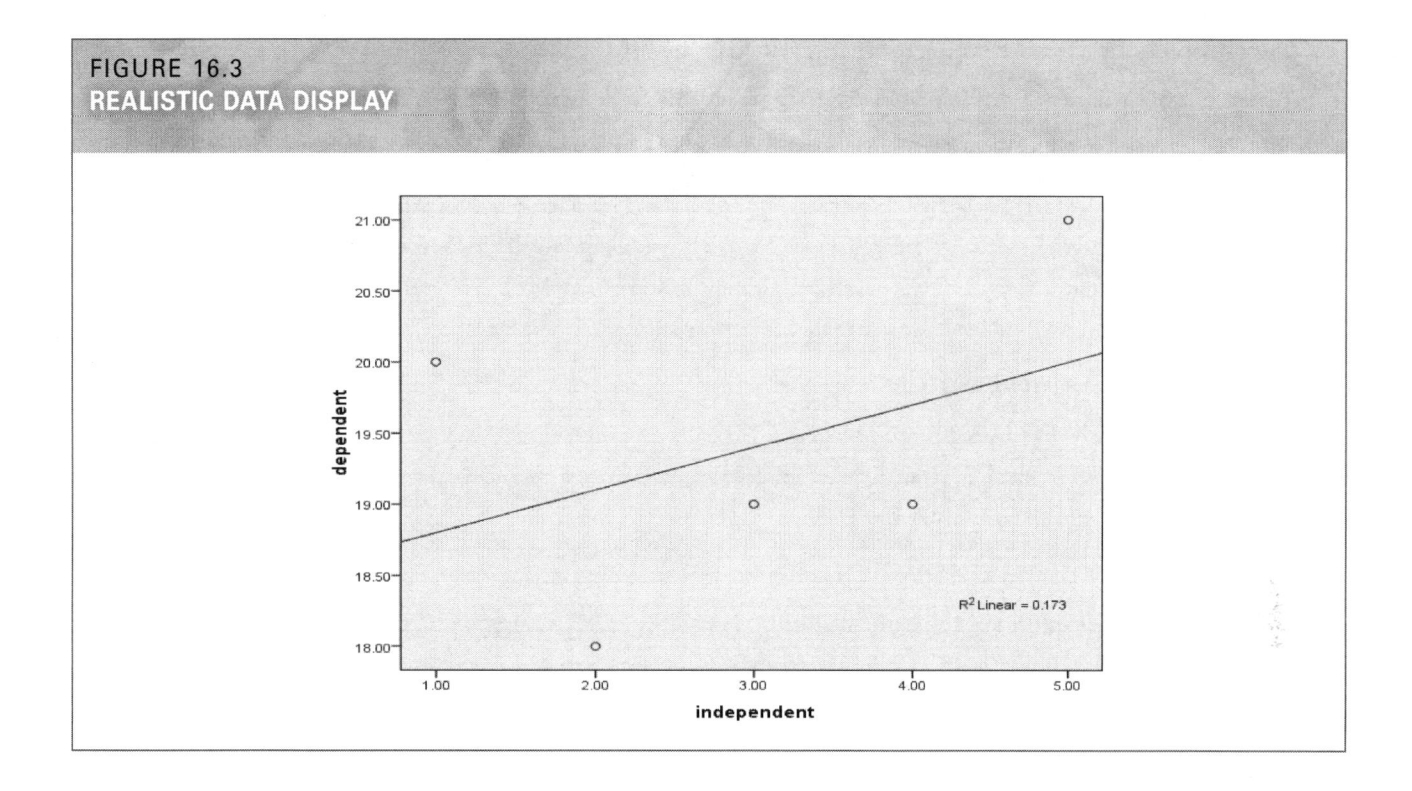

CORRELATION: THE IMPORTANCE OF MEASURING RELATIONSHIPS BETWEEN VARIABLES

FIGURE 16.3
REALISTIC DATA DISPLAY

Scatterplot 16.1 demonstrates a perfect positive correlation. The correlation is equal to +1.00. The X variable is the independent variable and is placed on the horizontal axis, and the Y or dependent variable is placed on the horizontal axis. In this example, there is a direct relationship, such that as each X variable leads directly to the same interval change in variable Y. When you have a perfect correlation, regardless of whether it is positive or negative, you can make perfect predictions about the values on the dependent variable.

Scatterplot 16.2 demonstrates a perfect negative correlation. As one can see, the slope of the line moves from the top left corner downward, toward the lower right corner of the graph. This is demonstrating a perfect negative correction of –1.00. This also demonstrates an inverse relationship, such that as X goes up, Y goes down or vice versa. In the case of this graph and the data presented as X or the independent variable goes up, the Y or dependent variable goes down.

Finally, scatterplot 16.3 demonstrates a more realistic data display. Notice where the data points exist on the graph. The regression line going through the middle of the data acts like a floating mean, and it demonstrates that, generally speaking, the correction is positive, as the line has a slight positive slope. The correlation is moderately positive, and its strength is +0.42 and is a moderately strong correlation. What this is stating is, generally speaking, as X or the independent variable goes up, so too does the Y or dependent variable.

CHAPTER 16

The previously described examples intentionally use hypothetical data points that did not pertain to any specific analysis as a way to help you understand how correlations work. Now that the preliminary discussion is out of the way, let's examine how correlation works using a specific data analysis.

Say you are examining the correlation between a person's height and weight. Given a group of 10 people, you measure each person's height and weight. After doing the statistical work, you determine that the correlation for height and weight for these 10 individuals is +0.70. What does this number mean? First, it is not a perfect correlation, but it is a strong correlation. Because it is a positive correlation, it is stating that, generally speaking, when variable X (height) goes up, variable Y (weight) also goes up; conversely, when variable X goes down, Y generally goes down. Positive relationships are direct relationships between the two variables under analysis.

Now say you want to examine the relationship between the amount of exercise an individual engages in and his or her cholesterol level. After examining a group of 50 individuals in a study, with a particular emphasis on the amount of exercise they engage in, and then conducting a blood test to examine the subjects' cholesterol level, you compute a correlation between exercise level and cholesterol level. The correlation that results is found to be −0.65, which is a strong negative correlation. Again, what does this result mean? First, you found a negative correlation, which means that, generally speaking, the lower the level on variable X (amount of exercise), the higher the level on variable Y (the person's cholesterol level). Conversely, the higher the level on variable X (amount of exercise), the lower the level found on variable Y (the person's cholesterol level). A negative relationship is an inverse relationship, such that when one variable goes up, the other generally goes down, and when one variable goes down, the other generally goes up.

Now suppose you're interested in examining satisfaction levels among your employees. You hypothesize that those who are paid higher salaries are much more satisfied in their work. You develop a satisfaction survey and pass it out to everyone. Upon receiving the completed surveys, you enter the data into a computer spreadsheet, compiling a satisfaction score from the survey on each employee and entering it with his or her respective salary.

Now, you hypothesized that the correlation would be fairly strong and positive. The results of the computation, however, demonstrate a correlation of +0.038. This correlation is surprising; it is slightly positive, but it is not far from 0. This correlation demonstrates that there apparently is not much of a relationship between satisfaction and salary.

What should we learn from these examples? For one, when conducting correlation research, you should avoid making *causal attributions*. In other words, correlation does not prove causation. For example, what

CORRELATION: THE IMPORTANCE OF MEASURING RELATIONSHIPS BETWEEN VARIABLES

if the correlation in the preceding example indicated a high association between satisfaction and salary? Could we say that a high salary led to greater satisfaction scores? Definitely not, because it's possible that those with higher job satisfaction scores have better jobs and receive higher salaries. Or it's possible that other variables may be playing a more important role—for example, those with higher education levels often will have better jobs and higher job satisfaction.

Similarly, does a low correlation mean job satisfaction is not appreciably influenced by salary? Definitely not, because it's possible that another, uncontrolled variable obscured the true relationship. Thus, with correlations, you must guard against attributing cause to any association or relationship that you may find among variables. Instead, you should stick with the facts as they are presented and avoid making causative attributions that correlations cannot support.

Partial correlation

One type of correlation that helps to control extraneous or confounding variables (variables that may contribute to spurious relationships) is *partial correlation*. Partial correlation gets its name from its control process, a process that partials out or controls for certain variables, while examining the correlation that exists among all the other variables.

The following is the formula for determining partial correlation:

$$r_{12 \cdot 3} \frac{r_{12} - r_{13}r_{23}}{\sqrt{(1 - r^2_{13})(1 - r^2_{23})}}$$

In the preceding formula:

- $r_{12} \cdot 3$ is the correlation between variables 1 and 2, holding 3 constant

- r_{12} is a correlation between variables 1 and 2

- r_{13} is a correlation between variables 1 and 3

- r_{23} is a correlation between variables 2 and 3

CHAPTER 16

Our earlier example examined how salary was related to job satisfaction. Remember that the example demonstrated almost a nonexistent correlation of 0.038. Now, for this example, let's say the relationship that was found between salary and job satisfaction was 0.578, a high correlation. Upon examining the data further, you decide to control for education and partial out the variables to obtain a better understanding of the relationship among them.

To do this you would use partial correlation. When examining the data, the computational results reveal the following:

- The correlation between salary and job satisfaction was 0.578

- The correlation between salary and education was 0.785

- The correlation between job satisfaction and education was 0.725

Now, using the partial correlation equation and plugging in the relevant data with the appropriate control factored into the equation, the magnitude of the correlation changes considerably.

$$r_{12 \cdot 3} = \frac{0.578 - (0.785)(0.725)}{\sqrt{(1 - 0.785^2)(1 - 0.725^2)}} = 0.021$$

The lower correlation results are related to the larger associations found between education and salary and education and job satisfaction. Education was playing an important role in the original relationship, but without controlling for education, as we did in the partial correlation, the impact that education had on the relationship was not obvious. The original correlation was influenced by a third variable: education. This would be important to you as a healthcare administrator, because say that after seeing the original correlation you were ready to introduce an across-the-board pay increase. But now, after seeing the results of the partial correlation, you decide to reconsider this wage increase, anticipating that if education is a prominent variable in work satisfaction, trying to affect worker attitudes by increasing everyone's pay may be fruitless.

17 Inferentially Based Statistical Procedures

The quantitative statistical procedures we have examined thus far are typically referred to as *descriptive* in nature. This is because they are based on examining issues by describing data that you have regarding the totality of a population. The *population* is the total number of elements you are examining. So, for example, if you were examining the wages of all the employees in your nursing facility, the population would be the wages of each worker in the facility. Or, if you were examining the efficacy of wound care, the population would be all the residents in the facility that have wounds that are being treated.

However, sometimes a healthcare administrator may need to examine a particular phenomenon, but he or she does not have knowledge of all of the elements that make up the entire population or even most of the population. This is when a *sample*—a subset of a hypothesized population—is taken and the results are generalized to the larger population with a fairly reasonable degree of accuracy. This is often referred to as *inferential statistical analysis*, because you are making inferences regarding potential phenomena concerning the population without knowing each and every element of the population. This happens, for example, when polls are conducted to examine political races, surveying perhaps 1,000 people and getting results that are close to what the larger U.S. voting population will cast in a forthcoming election. Sound inferential statistical analysis and sampling in this case would allow us to obtain results that are close to those that will be found on Election Day.

Hypotheses

Before we discuss inferential data analysis, we ought to revisit the topic of hypotheses. Earlier in the book, we discussed hypotheses as part of the scientific process. Here we will discuss hypotheses and hypothesis testing to acquaint you with common quantitative concepts that are often used to address hypothesis testing as it relates to quantitative methodology.

CHAPTER 17

The two types of hypotheses that are usually mentioned when performing quantitative/statistical procedures are the *null hypothesis* (usually abbreviated as H_0) and the *alternative hypothesis* (usually abbreviated as H_1).

The null hypothesis is often referred to as the hypothesis of no difference, meaning that it states that no statistically significant difference will be found. It also states that any difference that is found will be merely caused by chance.

Conversely, the alternative hypothesis is the hypothesis that states that what is found is something other than what was stated in the null hypothesis. For example, say you hypothesize that an employee's wages are important in terms of his or her level of job satisfaction. If you tested this and found that this was correct, you would reject the null hypothesis and accept the alternative hypothesis. However, if you evaluated the data and found that wage and job satisfaction were not significantly related, you would accept or fail to reject the null hypothesis.

Hypotheses can also state direction (one-tailed testing), or they can be nondirectional (two-tailed testing). For example, when a hypothesis states that medication X will be superior to medication Y, this test implies directionality, stating that X will be greater and will exceed the effect produced by Y. This is called a one-tailed test, because to obtain statistical significance, the statistical test results must meet and exceed a specific area on one side of the distribution. The following diagram demonstrates this:

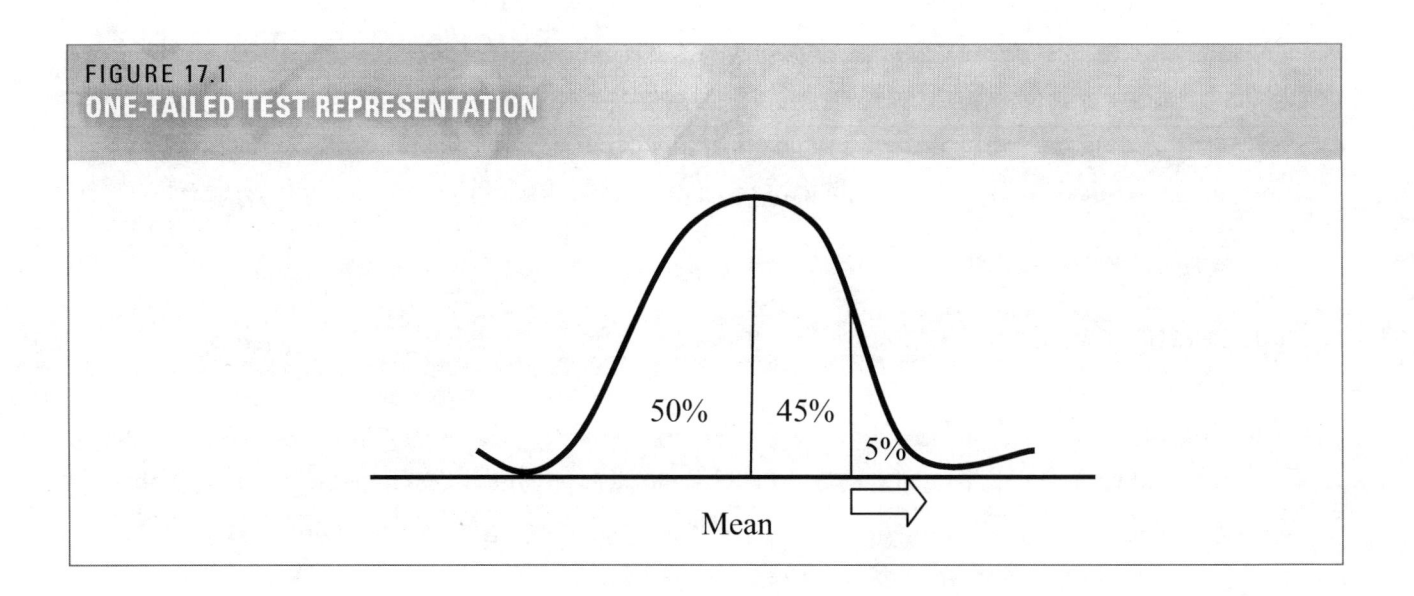

FIGURE 17.1
ONE-TAILED TEST REPRESENTATION

INFERENTIALLY BASED STATISTICAL PROCEDURES

This figure shows that for statistical significance to be achieved and for the null hypothesis to be rejected, the results must reach or exceed the line on the right side of the distribution, where the results meet and exceed 95% of the rest of the distribution. (Note, however, that this zone can vary. For example, if you want to meet a more stringent level, the line could be moved farther to the right, allowing for 99% of the distribution to be under the zone of statistical acceptance.)

Conversely, a hypothesis can be nondirectional, indicating a two-tailed test. The two-tailed test looks at both sides (tails) of the distribution to determine statistical significance. As an example, say you state that the results obtained from medication X will differ significantly from the results obtained from medication Y. The null hypothesis states that no difference will be found. Notice the nondirectional features of this hypothesis. It is not saying whether something is better or worse, superior or inferior; it is just stating that the results will be different. Again, if we use the distribution curve to illustrate this phenomenon, the zones for rejection of the null hypothesis now are at both ends, as the diagram below demonstrates.

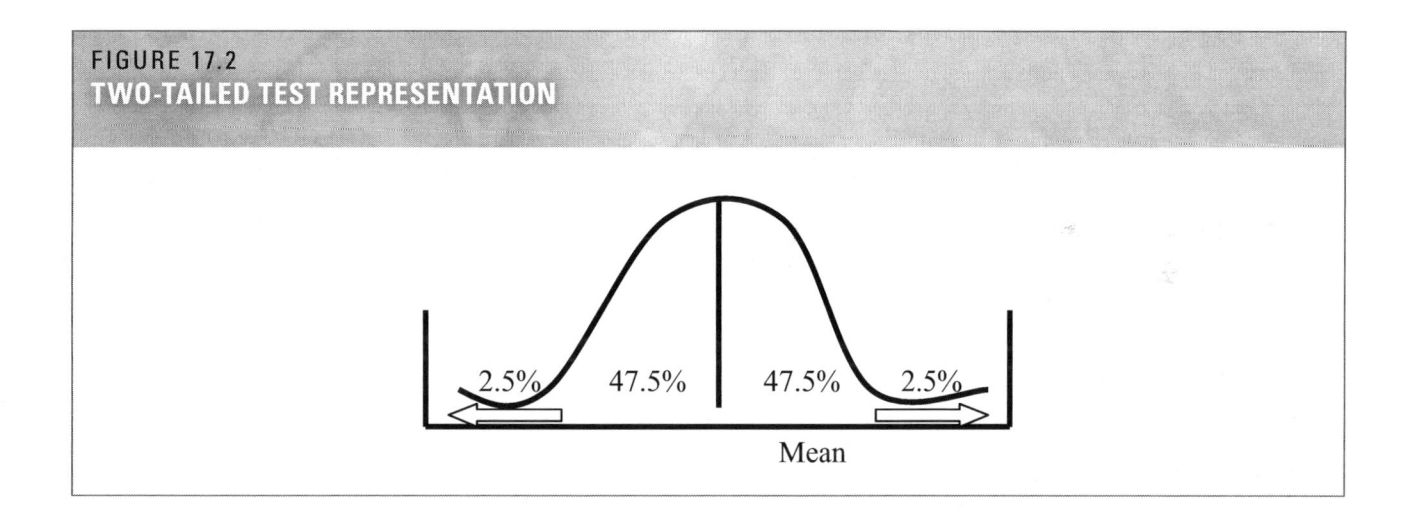

FIGURE 17.2
TWO-TAILED TEST REPRESENTATION

2.5% | 47.5% | 47.5% | 2.5%

Mean

Notice in the preceding figure where the zones of rejection for the null hypothesis exist. They are at both ends of the distribution—hence, they are two-tailed, and the results have to meet or exceed those two areas to achieve statistical significance. Again, as with the one-tailed test, you could introduce more stringent zones for rejecting the null hypothesis, and this would move each zone on each end of the distribution farther to the left and farther to the right.

What are these so-called zones that we have been discussing? Usually, when a person is going to engage in some type of inferential statistical analysis, not only will he or she determine the hypothesis and whether it will be directional, but also he or she will set a significance level, sometimes called an alpha (α) level. The alpha or

CHAPTER 17

significance level is the area in which the respective scores must fall to be considered statistically significant. The two most common statistical significance levels that are used are 0.05 and 0.01, often denoted as p = 0.05 and p = 0.01. (The p stands for probability.) With this in mind, our previous example indicates that the results obtained have met or exceeded the 0.05 or 0.01 zone for rejecting the null hypothesis. In other words, the results are strong, and we can expect them to appear by chance in only 5% or less or 1% or less of the cases.

To demonstrate this, say you decide to conduct research on Medicare receipts among various nursing facilities and you find out that facilities with more experienced MDS coordinators also have higher rates of Medicare reimbursement, proportionately speaking, due to greater knowledge of utilization of RUG categories that frequently are not utilized by less experienced MDS coordinators. You start with a directional hypothesis (a one-tailed test) stating that MDS coordinators with greater experience would also help to achieve greater Medicare revenue when compared to less experienced MDS coordinators. You then set the alpha level at 0.05.

The results would demonstrate an alpha of p = 0.035, which is significant at the 0.05 level. Therefore, you would reject the null hypothesis (H_0, or the hypothesis of no difference) and accept the alternative hypothesis (H_1), stating that the results were statistically significant and chance occurrences of such results could occur only 3.5 times or less in 100 occurrences.

Additional Tests

A few additional forms of statistical procedures used often are the one-sample z- and t-tests and the two-sample t-test.

The one-sample z-test

You use the *one-sample z-test* when you know your population mean and your population standard deviation. Say you are a healthcare administrator examining three facilities owned by your company and you are interested in examining how your company's long-term care facilities did compared to other facilities in your state on the basis of citations received from surveys. You know your state average or mean equals 9.2 citations with a standard error of the mean of 11.98. Your three facilities received an average of 8.8 citations. You would enter that information into the following formula:

$$Z = \frac{X - \mu}{\sigma x}$$

INFERENTIALLY BASED STATISTICAL PROCEDURES

The bar X stands for the sample mean; in this case it could represent the average of the company's three facilities. You would then subtract the population mean, which is the U-shaped symbol. Finally, you would divide that by the standard error of the mean. In this case, the standard error of the mean, or SEx, would be equal to dividing the standard deviation by the square root of N. N in this case would be the total number of nursing facilities in your state—say, 452. The square root of that equals 21.26. Now if the standard deviation is 11.98, that divided by 21.26 equals 0.5634, which is your standard error of the mean. By plugging in these numbers, you get the following:

$$Z = \frac{8.8 - 9.2}{0.5634} = -0.7099$$

This is a test of statistical significance. It states that your result is different from the population, and the results are statistically significant. We won't go into depth about probability sampling, but suffice it to say that statistical significance demonstrates a low likelihood that the results are based on chance and therefore the difference is an important difference. Usually, if this result were to be statistically significant at an alpha level of 0.05, a common standard for determining significance, it would have to meet or exceed a Z-score of 1.96, whether it is positive or negative. In this case, your company's facilities did well overall, compared to the state average, but your difference was not statistically significant. One final note: Do not confuse the z-test with the Z-score mentioned earlier, which places information into a standardized score.

The one-sample t-test

You would use the one-sample t-test when you know the population mean but you don't know the standard deviation for the population. The formula for employing the one-sample t-test is similar to that for the one-sample z-test, so we won't go into detail again.

However, note that today most mathematical procedures are performed on the computer, which gives us results much more quickly and efficiently than we can get when performing these calculations by hand. Nevertheless, healthcare administrators still need to understand what tests to employ, when to use them, and what the results mean. Placing data into a computer and running a quantitative procedure will produce results, but if you do not understand the results, they will be meaningless.

CHAPTER 17

Two-sample t-tests

Where the one-sample z- and t-tests examine single samples against known population data, the two-sample t-test compares the results of the mean of one sample against the mean of another sample to determine whether the means differ on a statistically significant level. There are two major types of two-sample t-tests: *independent* and *dependent*. In this section, we will discuss the independent t-test.

Let's say you are a managerial consultant for a corporation that owns 10 nursing homes. A company that sells pharmaceuticals is claiming to have a medication that is far superior to the product you are currently using for wound care. You decide to try this medication in one of your facilities. You randomly choose two of your facilities to be part of your sample—one facility will use the new product and the other will use your current product. You monitor both facilities for 60 days, applying measurements that would quantitatively identify wound healing. At the end of the 60 days, you examine the results, employing the following formula for an independent t-test:

$$T = \frac{M_1 - M_2}{\sqrt{\frac{S_1^2 + S_2^2}{N_1 + N_2}}}$$

Plugging in the numbers, M_1 is the mean for the nursing home using the new product and M_2 is the mean for the nursing home using the existing product that is subtracted from the first. This is divided by the square root of the sum of S_1^1 divided by N^1 for the first nursing home plus S_2^2 divided by N_2 for the second nursing home. Using this equation, the administrator will be able to determine whether nursing home number one using the new product is finding any statistically significant difference in the results of their wound care as compared to nursing home two, which is using the same wound care product it has been using.

Now let's say the first nursing facility was the one in which the new medication was used. In the first facility, 35 residents were evaluated for wound improvement using the standard treatment, and in the second facility, 32 residents were followed for wound care using the new medication. After 60 days, the mean for the instrument used to measure wound care and improvement was 32.580 for the first facility with a standard deviation of 4.30 and 18.859 for the second facility with a standard deviation of 1.25. For this

INFERENTIALLY BASED STATISTICAL PROCEDURES

example, the higher mean equates to greater improvement. The following are the following steps using the two sample t-tests.

M_1	M_2
32.580	18.859
4.30	1.25
35	32

Step one:

$M_1 - M_2 = 13.721$

Step two:

$$\frac{(4.30)^2}{1} + \frac{(1.25)^2}{1}$$

$18.49 + 1.56 = 20.05 = 4.48$

Step three:

$13.721 \div 4.48 = 3.06$

Was this a statistically significant difference? The t-score was 3.06, and you noticed that this was significant, even exceeding an alpha level of 0.01, which meant that this result could be influenced only by chance in 1 of 100 cases. Therefore, the result was impressive. So impressive, in fact, that you decide to sample two other nursing homes to see whether the new medication will continue to exhibit the same wound-healing efficacy. From this new data, you can decide whether to implement the new medication in all the corporation's nursing facilities.

ANOVA: A More Powerful Measuring Tool

In the preceding section, we examined how you can use t-tests to measure whether there is a significant difference between two sample means. In reality, often you have to examine differences between more than two means. Analysis of variance (ANOVA) is a more sophisticated measure you can use to examine whether there is a significant difference in a single independent variable found among the means of different grouping variables.

With this method, we are not just looking at two different means or grouping variables, as we did in the t-test, but rather three or more different means. For example, we could have extended the t-test to three

CHAPTER 17

nursing facilities, with one using the same protocol for wound care it has been using, another using a protocol that was stated as being superior to the existing protocol for wound care, and the third using the new medication that was purported as being the best form of treatment. In this case, you could sample these three nursing facilities with the aforementioned protocol to determine whether the mean scores for wound healing are better in one nursing facility over the others. With this hypothetical example, let us say the following results were obtained.

	Facility 1	Facility 2	Facility 3
Mean	18.45	18.97	35.89
Standard Deviation	1.98	2.01	1.035
F = 8.98 P = 0.001			

Using a one-way analysis of variance, that is, looking at only one independent variable (in this case, the medication), the results demonstrate statistical significance at the .001 level, which is a strong level of significance stating that the results obtained could be obtained only by chance in 1 case in 1,000. The formula for this is too involved to address, but the good news is that a good statistical program and even many spreadsheet programs can calculate this quickly. All you have to do is put the scores into the spreadsheet and run the analysis of variance.

Here's another example to help further explain this issue. Say you are interested in examining worker satisfaction, and you hypothesize that worker satisfaction will be related to higher levels of internal control, which was a concept discussed by Julian Rotter (1966) and basically states that a person whose locus of control is more internally based will feel greater control in his or her life; this subsequently transfers to the workplace. So, you feel that different employees, such as physicians, physical therapists, and laboratory technologists, will feel greater satisfaction due to greater autonomy and subsequently a greater locus of control. Conversely, employees with less internal control, such as housekeepers, nursing aides, and dietary personnel, will experience lower levels of job satisfaction.

You randomly sample 20% of the personnel in each department, using a locus of control scale and worker satisfaction scale as tools to conduct your research. You make the following distinctions: professional medical, nonprofessional medical, professional nonmedical, nonprofessional nonmedical, and administration. When you enter the data, your analysis demonstrates that there are significant differences in the rate of satisfaction and locus of control among the two groups and that those groups with higher mean scores

INFERENTIALLY BASED STATISTICAL PROCEDURES

on job satisfaction also have high mean scores on internal locus of control. In short, the ANOVA in this example states that the results are statistically significant at the 0.05 level.

Independent variables

ANOVA can also examine two or more independent variables. In the one-way ANOVA, only one independent variable was examined in both of the preceding examples. If we expand the ANOVA analysis and do a two-way ANOVA, we can examine two independent variables independently for statistical significance as well as an interaction between the two variables.

For example, say the CEO of your facility is concerned about a potential bias that may exist within the nursing department related to sex and minority status and how these two independent variables may influence promotion, especially to managerial nurse status. The CEO has heard about potential Title VII issues that may exist and decides to conduct an important study to see whether there is any justification for complaints in this area. The CEO states three hypotheses that may result:

- Males may be promoted more quickly and in greater numbers proportionately than females

- Nonminority status members may be promoted more quickly and in proportionately greater numbers than minority members

- Males and individuals with nonminority status will be promoted more quickly and in proportionately greater numbers

In conducting the study, the CEO randomly samples 250 nurses, making sure the sample represents the 10% of male nurses who work for the organization and therefore making the sample proportionate to the population. After examining the data acquired from human resources records and payroll, as well as an opinion questionnaire that was passed out, the CEO compiles the data and enters it into a computer for computational analysis. The following are the results the computer generated after the data from the study was entered:

	F-Ratio	Probability
Sex	3.987	0.049
Minority	3.995	0.0415
Sex * Minority	9.985	0.009

CHAPTER 17

The F-ratio is determined by calculating the mean variance between groups and dividing by the mean variance within groups, but it is not as simple as it sounds. However, the computer does this for you, so we do not need to go into detail. Suffice it to say that, generally speaking, the higher the F-ratio the greater the likelihood for statistically significant results. In examining the data analysis, the CEO notices that differences in promotion do indeed exist related to sex and minority status.

Both of these independent variables were significantly related to promotion, or lack of it, to managerial status, and both were significant at the 0.05 level. However, when combining sex and minority status, the F-ratio increased dramatically and statistical significance was found at the 0.01 level. Therefore, the CEO summarizes that one's sex and minority status are instrumental in terms of promotion within the corporation, with men and nonminority status nurses being promoted to higher levels with greater frequency. However, the CEO also finds that when one's sex and minority status are combined, the results take on even greater statistical significance, being significant at the 0.01 level with a nonminority male nurse considerably favored in being promoted to management status. The interaction between sex and minority status is important to note since it is not just sex, or minority status, but the interaction between the two variables that holds considerable impact as it relates to this issue.

These results are important to the CEO, as obtaining this type of information may help the CEO restructure the promotional system for nurses, address human resources policy, and maybe even institute some form of affirmative action policy to address the current promotional disparity found among nursing. This analysis can also help the CEO ward off any potential litigation that may be brought against the corporation for unfair promotional practices. It also helps to shed light on current promotional practices that may have some level of structural bias built in, with the results being found to be statistically significant.

INFERENTIALLY BASED STATISTICAL PROCEDURES

FIGURE 17.3
TABLE OF THE NORMAL DISTRIBUTION

| Z = (x-mean)/Standard Deviation |||||||||||
z	0	0.01	0.02	0.03	0.04	0.05	0.06	0.07	0.08	0.09
0	0	0.004	0.008	0.012	0.016	0.0199	0.0239	0.0279	0.0319	0.0359
0.1	0.0398	0.0438	0.0478	0.0517	0.0557	0.0596	0.0636	0.0675	0.0714	0.0753
0.2	0.0793	0.0832	0.0871	0.091	0.0948	0.0987	0.1026	0.1064	0.1103	0.1141
0.3	0.1179	0.1217	0.1255	0.1293	0.1331	0.1368	0.1406	0.1443	0.148	0.1517
0.4	0.1554	0.1591	0.1628	0.1664	0.17	0.1736	0.1772	0.1808	0.1844	0.1879
0.5	0.1915	0.195	0.1985	0.2019	0.2054	0.2088	0.2123	0.2157	0.219	0.2224
0.6	0.2257	0.2291	0.2324	0.2357	0.2389	0.2422	0.2454	0.2486	0.2517	0.2549
0.7	0.258	0.2611	0.2642	0.2673	0.2704	0.2734	0.2764	0.2794	0.2823	0.2852
0.8	0.2881	0.291	0.2939	0.2967	0.2995	0.3023	0.3051	0.3078	0.3106	0.3133
0.9	0.3159	0.3186	0.3212	0.3238	0.3264	0.3289	0.3315	0.334	0.3365	0.3389
1	0.3413	0.3438	0.3461	0.3485	0.3508	0.3531	0.3554	0.3577	0.3599	0.3621
1.1	0.3643	0.3665	0.3686	0.3708	0.3729	0.3749	0.377	0.379	0.381	0.383
1.2	0.3849	0.3869	0.3888	0.3907	0.3925	0.3944	0.3962	0.398	0.3997	0.4015
1.3	0.4032	0.4049	0.4066	0.4082	0.4099	0.4115	0.4131	0.4147	0.4162	0.4177
1.4	0.4192	0.4207	0.4222	0.4236	0.4251	0.4265	0.4279	0.4292	0.4306	0.4319
1.5	0.4332	0.4345	0.4357	0.437	0.4382	0.4394	0.4406	0.4418	0.4429	0.4441
1.6	0.4452	0.4463	0.4474	0.4484	0.4495	0.4505	0.4515	0.4525	0.4535	0.4545
1.7	0.4554	0.4564	0.4573	0.4582	0.4591	0.4599	0.4608	0.4616	0.4625	0.4633
1.8	0.4641	0.4649	0.4656	0.4664	0.4671	0.4678	0.4686	0.4693	0.4699	0.4706
1.9	0.4713	0.4719	0.4726	0.4732	0.4738	0.4744	0.475	0.4756	0.4761	0.4767
2	0.4772	0.4778	0.4783	0.4788	0.4793	0.4798	0.4803	0.4808	0.4812	0.4817
2.1	0.4821	0.4826	0.483	0.4834	0.4838	0.4842	0.4846	0.485	0.4854	0.4857
2.2	0.4861	0.4864	0.4868	0.4871	0.4875	0.4878	0.4881	0.4884	0.4887	0.489
2.3	0.4893	0.4896	0.4898	0.4901	0.4904	0.4906	0.4909	0.4911	0.4913	0.4916
2.4	0.4918	0.492	0.4922	0.4925	0.4927	0.4929	0.4931	0.4932	0.4934	0.4936
2.5	0.4938	0.494	0.4941	0.4943	0.4945	0.4946	0.4948	0.4949	0.4951	0.4952
2.6	0.4953	0.4955	0.4956	0.4957	0.4959	0.496	0.4961	0.4962	0.4963	0.4964
2.7	0.4965	0.4966	0.4967	0.4968	0.4969	0.497	0.4971	0.4972	0.4973	0.4974
2.8	0.4974	0.4975	0.4976	0.4977	0.4977	0.4978	0.4979	0.4979	0.498	0.4981
2.9	0.4981	0.4982	0.4982	0.4983	0.4984	0.4984	0.4985	0.4985	0.4986	0.4986
3	0.4987	0.4987	0.4987	0.4988	0.4988	0.4989	0.4989	0.4989	0.499	0.499
3.1	0.499	0.4991	0.4991	0.4991	0.4992	0.4992	0.4992	0.4992	0.4993	0.4993
3.2	0.4993	0.4993	0.4994	0.4994	0.4994	0.4994	0.4994	0.4995	0.4995	0.4995
3.3	0.4995	0.4995	0.4995	0.4996	0.4996	0.4996	0.4996	0.4996	0.4996	0.4997
3.4	0.4997	0.4997	0.4997	0.4997	0.4997	0.4997	0.4997	0.4997	0.4997	0.4998

18 The Time Value of Money and Forecasting

A penny saved is a penny earned, but that penny will not have the same value tomorrow that it has today or that it had a year ago. With that in mind, one important task that healthcare administrators often must address is the *time value of money*. This states that a dollar today will be worth more than a dollar in the future. As such, you as an administrator have to understand how an investment your company makes today will be influenced by varying levels of inflation as well as the current impact that a dollar has for investment. Therefore, you may often be interested in asking a couple of important questions:

1. What will the future value be of a present value amount?

2. What is the present value of an amount that is expected to yield future values?

Compounding and Discounting

You can answer the first question by *compounding*, which is determining future values of a present sum. You can answer the second question by *discounting*, which is the reverse of compounding and seeks to assess the present value of an anticipated future value.

Time value tables have been created to help with these calculations. They examine the time period of an investment in years along with the interest rate, either compounded or discounted. Your financial department would have access to these tables to help you make these calculations, and a couple of these have been included at the end of this chapter as well. That being said, it is not as difficult as it sounds. You can estimate the future value of an investment by using the following formula:

$$FV \text{ (future value)} = (\$1 \times r)^n$$

This says that the future value of an investment is equal to the current dollar amount ($1), multiplied by the discount rate (r), which is found in the present value table based on (n), which is the number of years until the payment of the investment. For example, the future value of $1 invested at 10% (discount rate) for one year (n) is equal to $1.10.

What if you were interested in the future value of $500,000 invested at 8% for five years? The formula would look like this:

$$FV = (\$500,000 \times 1.46933)^5 = \$734,665$$

You would find the discount rate of 1.46933 in the time value tables at the end of this chapter. You'd find the value of 1.46933 by looking at the row at the five-year point in the table and moving horizontally to where it intersects at 8%.

Future Investments

What if you want to know the value of a future investment in current or present value dollars? For example, in the preceding example, what if you paid $734,665 for an investment that would be worth the same amount in five years? Unfortunately, this would not be consistent with the term investment.

For example, say that as a long-term care administrator, you want to invest in a large-scale renovation of the therapy department by adding more extensive equipment to provide better and more expansive physical and occupational services. The investment in the project over the next two years at 8% interest will add an expected increase in revenue of $1,500,000.

The present value is based on the following equation:

$$PV = FV_n [1/(1 + i)]^n$$
$$PV = \$1,500,000 [1/(1 + 0.08)]^2$$
$$PV = \$1,500,000 \times 0.8573 = \$1,285,950$$

In the preceding equation, (n) equals the number of years of the investment and (i) is the interest (discount) rate. Given that the facility is investing $200,000 for renovation for the therapy area, with a projected increase in revenue over two years of $1,500,000, the facility should not invest any more than the present value amount noted in the preceding figure. However, because the $200,000 investment is far from the present value of $1,285,950, and because the investment will be exceeded by revenues over the next two years that are 7.5 times greater than the investment, the project appears viable.

THE TIME VALUE OF MONEY AND FORECASTING

Before engaging in a project, many healthcare administrators apply the time value of money concept to evaluate the net present value (NPV), which examines the positive and negative cash flows that may exist over the life of an investment, to determine whether they should enter such an investment. However, the value of money is not static, and often a project that is entered into does not demonstrate an immediate return on investment. Furthermore, the time value of money prevents a project from frequently being analyzed on a linear basis. For example, in Chapter 4 we discussed the payback period ratio, which views the payback period as a constant and does not evaluate for time changes in the value of money. The NPV examines whether, after discounting for the time value of money for each year involved in the investment, the final cumulative time values still present criteria for undertaking the project or investment.

Let's modify the preceding example of the refurbished therapy room and determine whether such an investment will be productive. In this case, you are faced with two alternatives: keeping the current therapy room with no changes, or renovating the therapy room, leading to possible expansion of services and increasing revenue from this revenue center.

You put together a three-year strategic budget and operational plan, which includes projections for therapy as it currently exists versus whether it is renovated, projected revenue from both alternatives over the next three years, and what the cost of each will be, as well as estimating the NPV to determine whether services in this area should be expanded or left as they are. In this example, you feel that by investing $200,000, the facility will increase its revenue in this area by almost $1 million over a three-year period. The initial investment with cash flow is determined for both alternatives, and the projections are as follows:

Anticipated Revenue for Both Alternatives over a Three-Year Period

Time Period	Current	Renovations
0	0	($200,000)
1	$1,000,000	$800,000
2	$1,100,000	$1,400,000
3	$1,200,000	$1,900,000

Discounted Cash Flow and Net Present Value over Three Years at 10% Interest

Current	Discounted	Renovations	Discounted
			$(200,000)
$1,000,000	(0.9091) $909,100	$800,000	(0.9091) $727,280
$1,100,000	(0.8264) $909,040	$1,750,000	(0.8264) $1,446,200
$1,200,000	(0.7513) $901,560	$1,900,000	(0.7513) $1,427,470
	NPV = $2,719,700		NPV = $3,400,950

Finance, Budgeting & Quantitative Analysis: A Primer for Nursing Home Administrators

CHAPTER 18

We can see that given the projected revenue, the renovations will be increased by almost $1.2 million. However, when the time value of money is figured for each of the three years based on projected revenue, minus the initial investment, the renovations will lead to an anticipated $681,250 increase in revenue over the next three years. Because the NPV is greater than it would be if you kept the therapy area as is, this investment is justified. If the NPV was less than the current situation, it would not make sense to enter into the investment. In this case, you would decide to enter into the investment based on the NPV calculations.

Break-Even Analysis

Now let's say you are a healthcare administrator interested in starting an Alzheimer's unit. Within your geographic area, there is a need for such a unit. However, it would require a considerable level of construction to add on to the existing building as well as provide life safety updates that are consistent with current codes. Furthermore, specially trained staff, added wages, and specially designed areas will need to be considered to assist with the special needs of this population. Will this be a profitable business endeavor, or will you enter into something that will not be profitable? Furthermore, how many residents will the unit need to service just to break even financially?

With many investments there are fixed costs, which are known and will not fluctuate, and there are variable costs, which have a greater level of variability. In this example, you know most of the costs and what percentage of those costs is fixed and variable. However, what point does the facility have to meet just to break even? This is a critical question not just in healthcare but also in all businesses.

The break-even analysis uses a formula that is then graphed to demonstrate the break-even point a facility has to meet as well as where it loses or makes money. The break-even formula is as follows:

Break-Even Analysis = Fixed Costs + Variable Costs

Be = F + V

In this example of the new Alzheimer's wing, the fixed costs are projected at $1 million, and the variable costs are projected at 40% of the break-even resident days. The following would be the estimated break-even point.

$$Be - 40\%Be = \$1,000,000$$
$$60\%Be = \$1,000,000$$
$$Be = \frac{\$1,000,000}{0.60} = \$1,667,000 \text{ (rounded)}$$

THE TIME VALUE OF MONEY AND FORECASTING

Therefore, to break even, the new wing has to accrue $1,667,000 for the year. Anything over that amount would be profit, and anything under that amount would be loss. This break-even analysis helps you understand what you need to achieve on paper before entering into this project.

The break-even point we just calculated is based on resident days. Therefore, if the facility is sitting well in the market and will attract many residents, it will do well. However, if another facility enters the picture and vies for these residents, it can cause a competitive marketplace, possibly precluding your facility from reaching the break-even point. The following is the break-even graph demonstrating what the equation has already delineated.

From this, you can determine that the occupancy rate, based on the fixed costs allocated for each patient in the proposed 30-bed Alzheimer's unit, will have to be maintained at 86.67% occupancy over the year to be around the break-even point.

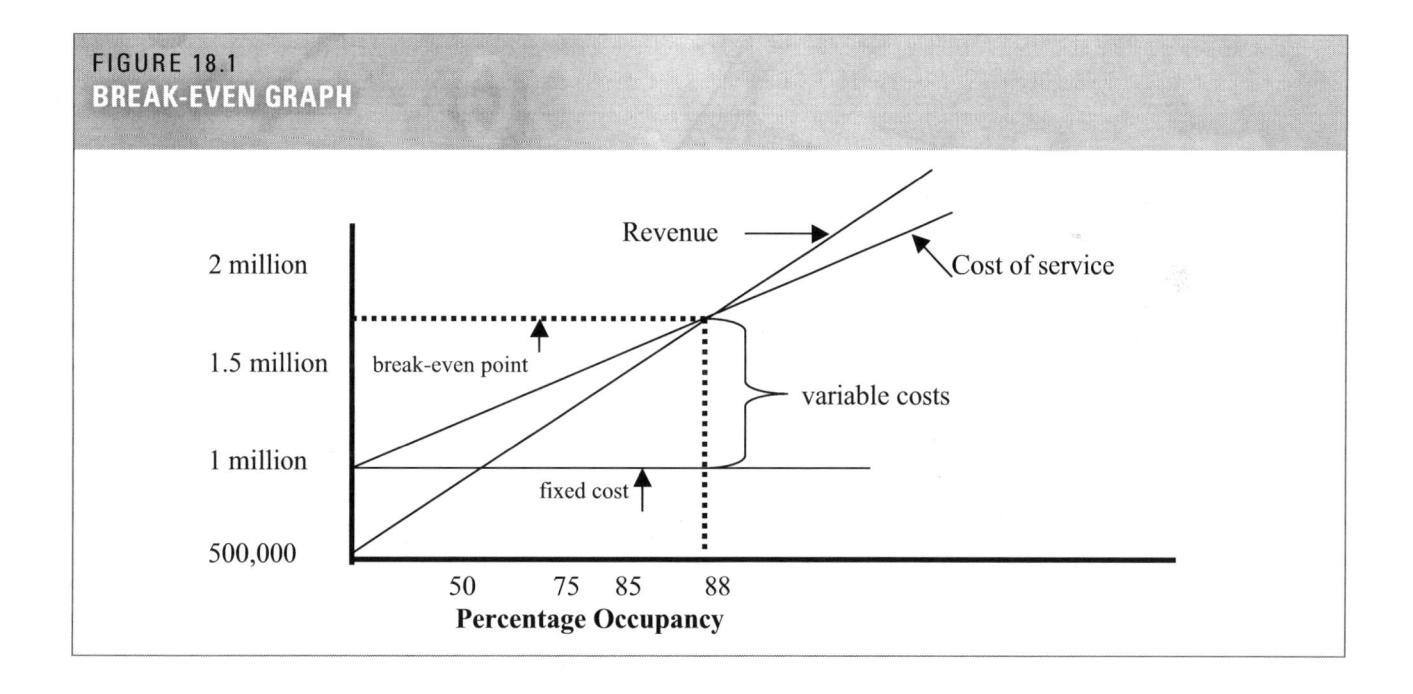

FIGURE 18.1
BREAK-EVEN GRAPH

CHAPTER 18

Forecasting: Looking Into the Future

Forecasting is an approach that is used to anticipate future events. What will our return be over the next quarter? How will inflation impact car and home sales? How will new legislation impact reimbursement for emergency services? All these questions are asking for some type of prediction. In other words, given these changes—the independent variable(s) x; x and y; or x, y, and z—how will they influence the future of the dependent variable Y' (read as Y prime)?

Often, experts will come together to give their "opinions" of what they anticipate the future holds given current changes in certain independent variables. This is a type of forecasting based on expert opinions, or what Seidel, Gorsky, & Lewis (1995) called *genius forecasting*, referring to the use of expert opinions to give information about the future. However, this type of approach is not very scientific, as it fails to base its conclusions on three important tenets of scientific inquiry: systematization, objectivity, and empiricism. Therefore, healthcare researchers and administrators prefer to use approaches that lend themselves to a greater scientific basis, using mathematical models to help forecast future events with a greater degree of certainty than often is found with pure opinions.

Numerous types of forecasting approaches can be employed for healthcare administration purposes. However, none of them is pristine or totally infallible. Forecasting always holds some degree of potential error. Random error that often occurs just due to chance circumstances can affect results significantly and is hard to control. Systematic error, however, is much more controllable. This is error that results from an impaired design quality, often due to the healthcare administrator and other researchers not thinking about the research well in advance and just trying to plug numbers into a computer.

Frequently, people become so fascinated with doing mathematical analysis and completing a sophisticated mathematical procedure that they gloat over their accomplishment, thinking they have accomplished something marvelous. Yet, they may have used a procedure that was inappropriate, and the results obtained are misleading due to the systematic error involved. Furthermore, what they may think they found in their research may not have any logical connection among the independent and dependent variables. This section will demonstrate some common forecasting methods that healthcare administrators often use.

THE TIME VALUE OF MONEY AND FORECASTING

Forecasting guidelines

There are some important guidelines to be aware of when conducting forecasting. Seidel, Gorsky, & Lewis (1995) state that the following guidelines should be followed without exception:

- Plot the data first.

- Follow a one-third rule of thumb whereby a forecast does not exceed one-third of the historical data that it is relying on for information. For example, if you are using six months of historical data to determine a forecast, generally speaking the forecast should not be for more than two months.

- Be conservative. This is the same rule that is followed when doing accounting and financial work. In other words, err on the side of pessimism.

Extrapolation is taking something that is known and inferring something that is not known. This is often the essence of what is meant by *prediction* and *forecasting*. I will demonstrate a couple of different forecasting methods here: one that deals with average change and one that deals with confidence intervals.

Extrapolation

Extrapolation based on average change examines the change of the independent variable to estimate or forecast the dependent variable. Extrapolation based on average change to forecast is based on the following formula:

> **Forecast Y = mean + (midpoint × average change)**

Given the preceding formula, the mean is equal to the summation of X, the independent variable, divided by N, or the number of observations. The midpoint is a type of median, but in this case it is the middle-most point in the number of observations. For example, if you were examining census data for the past three months to predict the upcoming month, you may have a census of 86%, 88%, and 90%, but you would look at only the three observations, with the midpoint equaling 2. You'd find the average change by taking each of the cases representing variable X, subtracting the mean from each, adding the total changes, and dividing the total by the number of observations.

CHAPTER 18

An example will help to illustrate this concept. Say that as a long-term care administrator, you are interested in forecasting the census for the upcoming month of May. During the first four months of the year, the census was as follows: 87%, 89%, 89%, and 91%. First you would plot the data on a graph to help provide a visual depiction of the data.

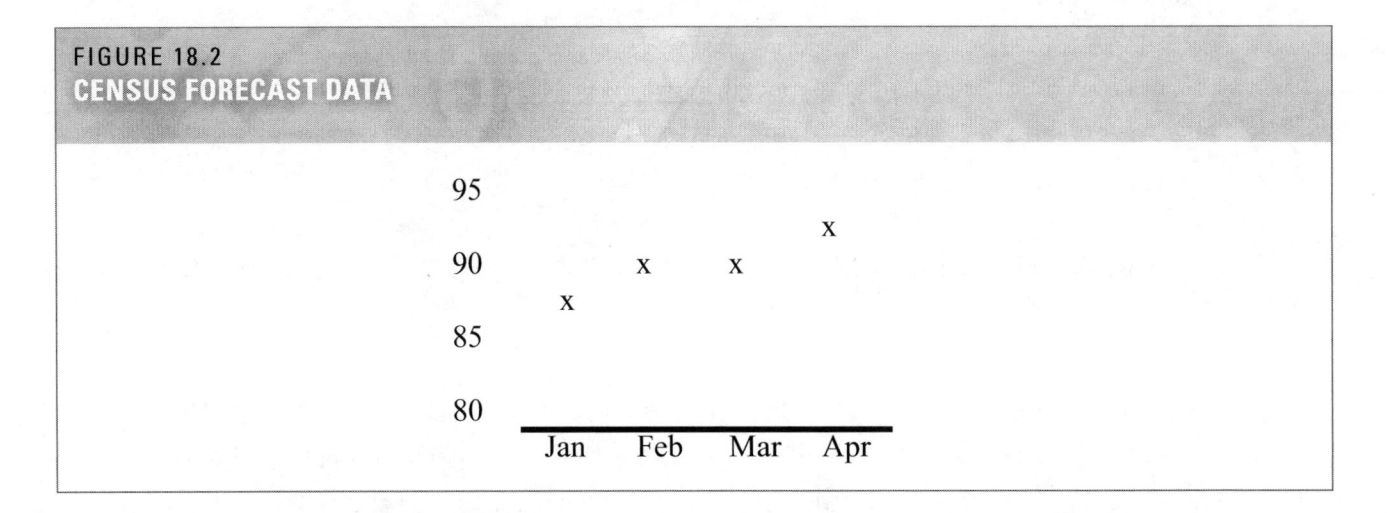

FIGURE 18.2
CENSUS FORECAST DATA

```
95
                              x
90         x    x
     x
85

80 ─────────────────────
    Jan  Feb  Mar  Apr
```

The data in the figure demonstrate a positive slope: For the first four months, there was an increase in the census. Now you must interpret the forecasted census for May based on the extrapolation technique for average change. So, you place the information into a table, as shown here:

Month	Census	Changes
January	87	
February	89	2
March	89	0
April	91	2
Mean:	89	Average Change = 4/3 = 1.33

(average change = sum of scores ÷ periods of change)

Midpoint = 2 + 3/2 = 2.5

(Midpoint fomula for midpoint is number X (in this case months) + 1 ÷ 2)

Forecasted Census for May = 89 + (2.5 x 1.33)
Forecasted Census for May = 92.325 or 92% (rounded)

THE TIME VALUE OF MONEY AND FORECASTING

These results demonstrate a forecasted census of 92%. However, this has to be taken with some caution. The month of May is a spring month, and that may demonstrate different census levels than winter months. So, you might want to look at the month of May for the past three to five years. However, five years can also be a problem given the time period. Therefore, another alternative may be to examine the census for the month of April, plus the months of April and May for the previous two years.

Regardless of the method you use, it's important to remember that possible permutations can cause misleading results and that no one method can lead to superior results. It is up to you to not engage in cursory decisions and instead to consider which method is best and what criteria to use. Remember, it is important in any type of quantitative analysis to eliminate as much error from the systematic realm as possible.

Extrapolation based on confidence intervals

Another method you can use to forecast is extrapolation based on confidence intervals. This method provides you with an area in which the forecasted score may fall, rather than a specific score as in the previous example. Before we get into the details, we should briefly discuss the confidence interval.

A confidence interval provides an area within which a score will fall. It also provides an interval of confidence, such as 95%, which measures how convinced we are that a score will fall within those given parameters. As an example, say you are interested in sampling nursing homes in your county to determine what the average census was, and you want to evaluate your facility in relation to this data. The census data for the randomly sampled nursing facilities over three months had a mean of 88%. The standard deviation was 2.02. To figure out the confidence interval, you first have to calculate the standard error of the mean, which you determine with the following formula:

$$SE\,\bar{x} = \frac{S}{\sqrt{N}} \text{ or } \frac{2.02}{2.828} = 0.71$$

If the standard deviation (S) equals 2.02 and the number of nursing facilities (N) examined was 8, the square root of 8 equals 2.828, which divided into 2.02 equals a standard error of 0.71. If you multiply the standard error by 1.96, that gives you the parameters for estimating 95% confidence in your results falling within the given confidence interval. If you multiply the standard error by 2.58, that provides you with a 99% confidence interval and a 99% confidence level that your results will fall within this interval.

CHAPTER 18

Using the aforementioned mean of 88%, if you multiply 1.96 by the standard error of 0.71, you get 1.39. Let's examine how that works to establish a confidence interval at a 95% level of confidence.

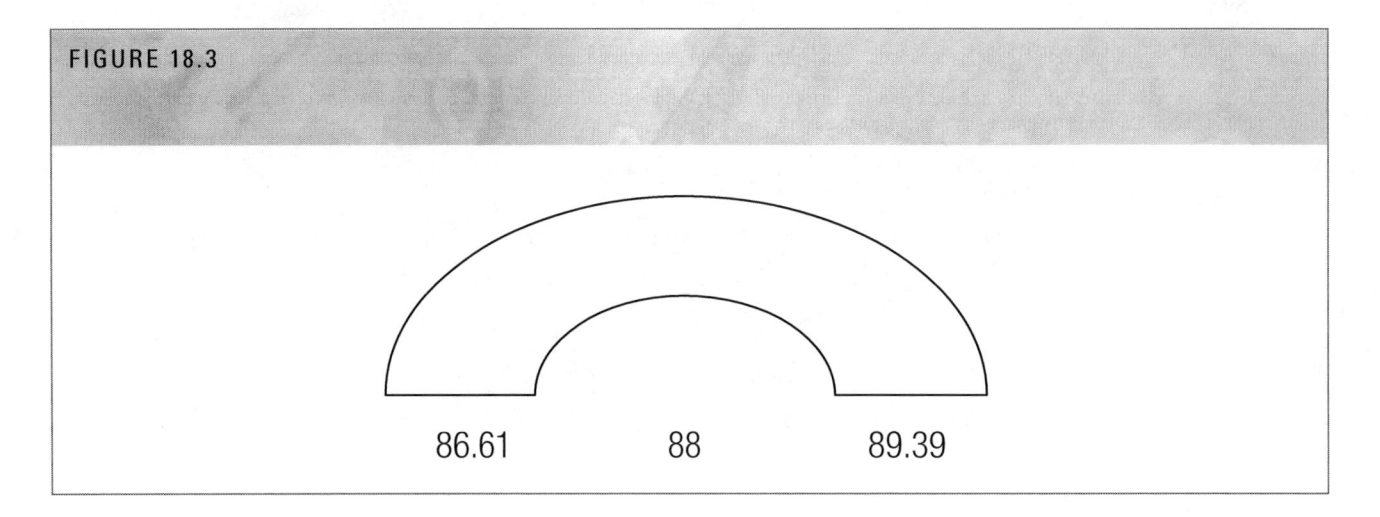

FIGURE 18.3

86.61   88   89.39

The interval between 86.61 and 89.39 is the confidence interval for a level of confidence at 95%. The 1.39 that you obtained from multiplying the 1.96 by the obtained standard error is added to the mean of 88 to obtain the upper limit, in this case 89.39, and is subtracted from the mean to get the lower limit, in this case 86.61. In this example, you are interested in comparing your nursing home's average census for a three-month period with the other nursing facilities in your county. You did not sample the entire county, just eight nursing facilities. But you did randomly sample these eight and you came away with an average census of 88%. You are 95% confident that the population mean falls somewhere between 86.61 and 89.39. Furthermore, your nursing home had an average census of 90%. Therefore, you can assume that, based on 95% confidence as it relates to the larger population, which is the entire county your nursing home resides in, your facility is doing well, comparatively speaking, with its census.

If you wanted to express a greater level of confidence, you could determine the confidence intervals at 99% confidence, which would be 2.58 × standard error (0.71), and this sets the confidence intervals at the mean of 88 ± 1.83. This now sets the upper limit at 89.83 and the lower limit at 86.17. You can see that this expands the confidence interval, providing greater assurance that the results you obtained from your sample approximate the population mean within a given confidence range.

To move forth with forecasting on the extrapolation based on confidence intervals, we can use the same example of forecasting the potential census for the month of May. Again, the first thing to do is to graph the data. The next step is to compute the standard deviation for the data. This is illustrated using the census data previously shown with the standard deviation calculation.

THE TIME VALUE OF MONEY AND FORECASTING

Month	Census	(X – M)	(X – M)²
January	87	–2	4
February	89	0	0
March	89	0	0
April	91	+2	4
Mean	89	0	8

$$\frac{\sqrt{(X-M)^2}}{N} = 8/4 = 2$$

$$SD = \sqrt{2} = 1.41$$

Now the Standard Error of the Mean can be calculated

$$SE\,\bar{x} = \frac{S}{\sqrt{N}} = \frac{1.41}{2} = 0.71$$

Now the 95% Confidence Interval = 1.96 x 0.71 = 1.39

Given this information, we can state that the mean is 89% with a standard error of the mean of 0.71. When the standard error is multiplied by 1.96 to achieve a 95% confidence interval, the result is 1.39. Just as in the example of confidence intervals earlier, we take the mean score, 89%, and first add and then subtract 1.39 from it to obtain the upper and lower limits of the confidence interval. This establishes a confidence interval where you can be 95% confident that the next month's census will fall. This being the case, with a level of confidence of 95%, the following interval is established.

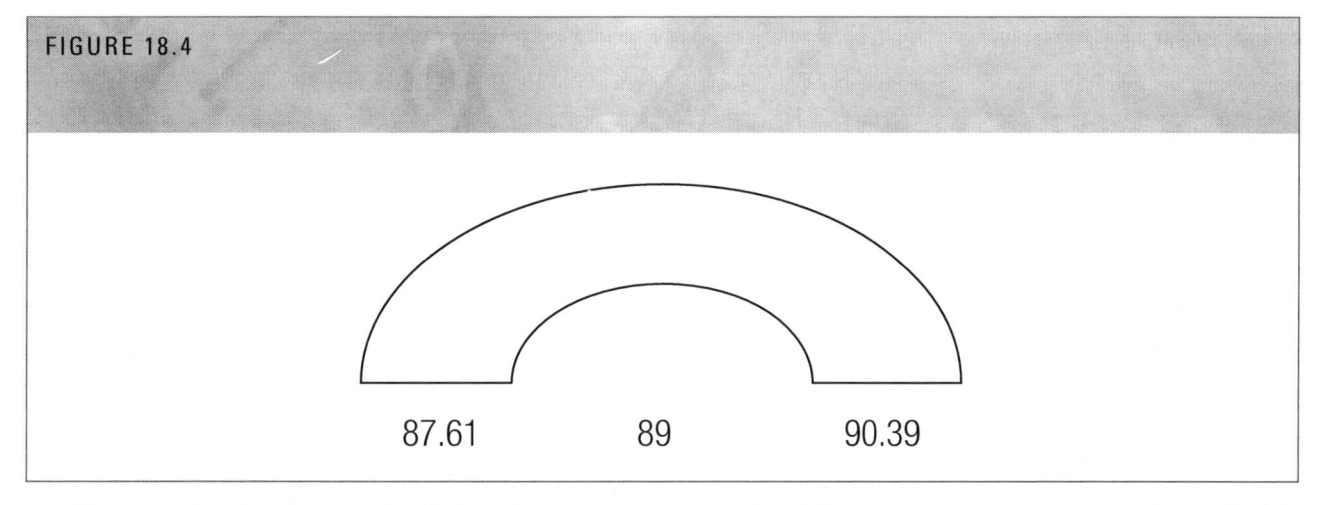

FIGURE 18.4

87.61   89   90.39

This says that for the month of May, the census is projected to fall within an interval ranging from 87.61% to 90.39% and that you are 95% confident that the census will fall somewhere within this interval for the month of May. Notice that this forecast provides an estimated interval based on a level of confidence, which differs from the point estimate based on average change seen in the previous forecasting method.

CHAPTER 18

If you needed greater assurance of where the upcoming month's census would fall, you could use a 99% confidence level. In doing this, you would take the standard error of 0.71 and instead of multiplying it by 1.96, you would now multiply it by 2.58:

> 99% confidence interval = 2.58 × 0.71 = 1.83

Again, this increases the interval, and in doing so, it also increases your level of confidence that the forecasted May census will fall somewhere between the upper and lower levels.

The following diagram shows that the intervals have increased at a level of 99% confidence. The 99% confidence intervals go from a low of 87.17% to a high of 90.83%. This is stating that you have gained greater assurance that May's census will fall within this interval. In other words, you are 99% confident that the census will fall somewhere within this interval.

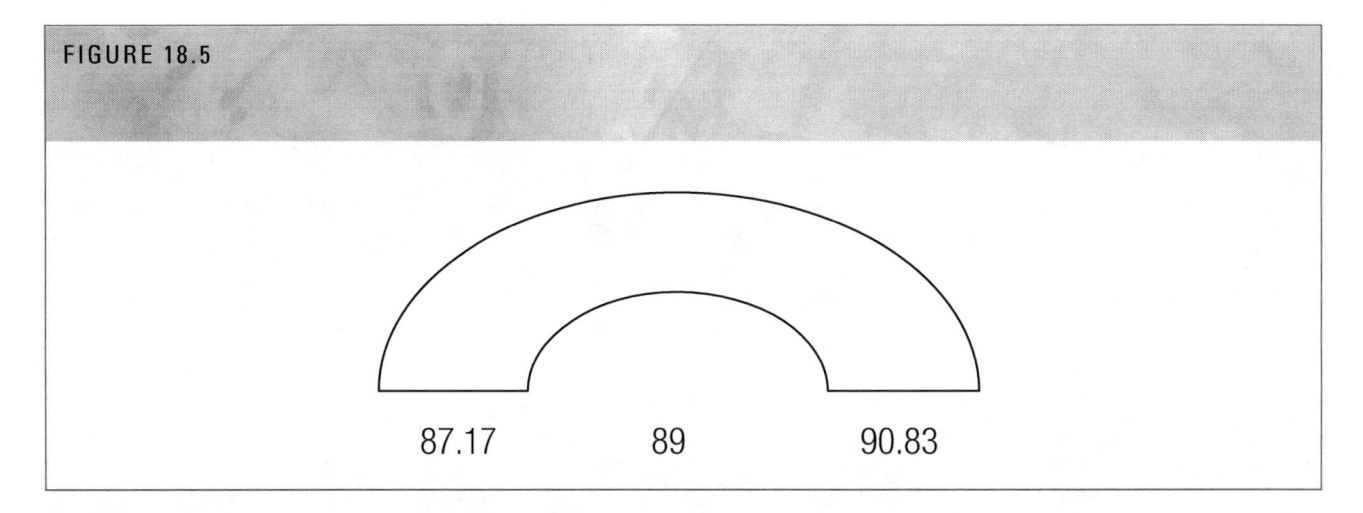

FIGURE 18.5

87.17   89   90.83

Extrapolation based on sensitivity analysis

Sometimes you may have changes within or outside your facility's environment that can introduce change into your forecast. *Sensitivity analysis* helps the administrator manipulate independent variables due to change that exists and may have an important impact on the dependent variable (Seidel, Gorsky, & Lewis, 1995). In other words, sensitivity analysis can help you anticipate future events that may occur due to some type of change, either expected or unexpected, and leading to one or more possible permutations that may affect the dependent variable.

Continuing with the census example, now say that you would like to forecast your census for the upcoming month of May. However, a nursing home within the relevant geographic area will be closing at the end of April, and this may have an important impact on your census.

THE TIME VALUE OF MONEY AND FORECASTING

You know you must examine the situation well because you will need to anticipate how much supplies and staffing you will need during the next month. You also know that the forecasted census, holding all things constant and not considering the closing of the other nursing home, predicts a May census of 92%. This is based on the first four months of the year, which have a mean of 89% and a standard error of 0.71. In addition, you note that there are two feeder hospitals in the area and three other nursing homes, all within a 5-mile radius of each other.

In compiling data from admissions on acceptance and denial of nursing home placement by prospective family members, you compute that approximately 40% of the referrals among the three nursing facilities end up coming to your facility. Also, you examine admissions or in-migration into the facility, as well as out-migration due to mortality, short-term respite, or rehabilitative improvement leading to discharge. Given all this information, you project that the closing of the facility, coupled with the possible placement of some residents in your facility, as well as factoring in hospital transfers and home admissions, minus the loss of residents due to mortality, short-term stay, or rehabilitative improvement, will lead to a census increase of approximately 5% of the initial projection for the month of May. This now will lead to a forecasted census for May of 96.6%.

Extrapolation based on the concept of moving averages

It also can be helpful to use the concept of moving averages (Seidel, Gorsky, & Lewis, 1995) in forecasting. This concept examines the changing averages over a period of time that precedes the period to be forecasted, and it examines the changing variability over these periods. It attempts to select a period that has the least variability, subsequently leading to a greater ability to forecast a specific variable for a specific period.

To further examine this concept, we will continue to use our earlier census example. Again, the first thing you would do is to plot the data on a graph. The next step is to calculate the n-period and the moving averages that are associated with the n-periods. An n-period has to always be greater than 1. The n-period is the look-back period for helping to calculate the moving averages. It works as follows:

Month	Census	n = 2	n = 3	n = 4
January	87			
February	89			
March	89	88		
April	91	89	88.33	
May	87	90	89.67	89

Mean = 88.6

CHAPTER 18

For the n = 2 period, notice that the first two rows have no values. This is because you need to start with the month of March to have an adequate two-period (n) look-back (February and January). If November or December was included in this data, the n = 2 could have started with the month of January. The n = 3 and n = 4 are the same. For n = 3, the first month that a moving average could be calculated for given the data and the three-month look-back period is April. For n = 4, the first month that a moving average could be calculated for is the month of May, given the need for a four-month look-back period.

The next step is to determine the forecast error. The forecast error is equal to the actual obtained value minus the forecasted value:

$$FE = (Actual\ value - Forecasted\ value)$$

This is placed as a column next to each n-period. For each forecasted error, an absolute deviation and a mean absolute deviation are calculated. The n-period with the lowest mean absolute deviation, indicating the n-period with the least variability, would be the n-period that would be used in forecasting future results.

Month	Census	n = 2	FE	n = 3	FE	n = 4	FE
January	87						
February	89						
March	89	88	1				
April	91	89	2	88.33	2.67		
May	87	90	-3	89.67	−2.67	89	−2
Absolute deviation			6		5.34		2
Mean absolute deviation			2		2.67		2

The preceding example is simple; all numbers were rounded, and only a few months were used. However, it provides enough information to understand the concept. First, the absolute deviation is the summation (in absolute value) of the forecast error. You disregard the signs found in the forecast error and sum each forecast error column. The mean absolute deviation is the absolute deviation divided by the number of observed n-periods that were calculated. For example, in the n = 2 column, three periods or numbers of observations were calculated; in the n = 3 column, two were calculated, and in the n = 4 column, one was calculated. The final step is to observe which of the mean absolute deviations demonstrates the least variation. In this example, the n = 2 period and n = 4 period both have mean absolute deviations of 2.0, demonstrating the lowest variances. However, since there are two FE categories that share the same mean absolute deviation, choose the one that represents the greatest number of scores. In this example, it would be the n = 2 category that examines three scores rather than the n = 4 category that only examines one. This, in turn, would be the n-period that would be used to forecast any further census data. If you were interested in forecasting June's census, given your knowledge that the n = 2 period would hold the least variance and therefore the possibility for greater levels of predictive accuracy, the forecasted census for June would be equal to the following:

> June Moving Average for Census = 87 (May) + 91 (April)/2 = 89

Using Regression Analysis as a Source of Forecasting

Regression analysis helps to predict and forecast many forms of phenomena. It is used frequently in education, business, and insurance, among other areas, and healthcare administrators will also make frequent use of this important technique. It is an extension of correlation, which we examined earlier. Again, as with most other quantitative methods we've examined in this chapter, computerized spreadsheets or statistical programs are the best and most efficient means to calculate this data analysis. This section will examine forecasting using regression analysis and only two variables. However, often more than one predictor (independent) variable needs to be taken into consideration to adequately evaluate the criterion (dependent) variable. This is when multiple regression analysis needs to be used. This section will concentrate on examining bivariate or two-variable analysis involving a single predictor variable forecasting a criterion variable.

Bivariate regression analysis

Bivariate regression analysis attempts to predict or forecast what a specific criterion variable will be, given knowledge of some predictor variable. Many former algebra students will recognize the following equation used to describe a straight line:

$$Y = aX + b$$

This equation demonstrates that Y', which is the criterion or forecasted variable, read as Y prime, is equal to the slope multiplied by the predictor variable, with b or the Y-intercept added to the product. The slope is equal to the change in Y divided by the change in X, often referred to as the rise divided by the run.

CHAPTER 18

The letter b is the Y-intercept, and it refers to the value of Y at the point where X equals 0, or the point at which the line crosses the y-axis.

To better understand this concept, consider this example. Say you are interested in forecasting the expected number of admissions for the upcoming month based on the number of referrals your facility receives. You examined the data for the past nine months and noticed that each month had varying levels of referrals, but when you rounded the average number of referrals, it came to approximately 30 referrals. You entered the exact number of referrals that the facility received for each of the past nine months. You also entered with each month the number of admissions the facility obtained from the referrals. As you would expect, the actual admissions that resulted from the actual number of referrals were different. When you entered this data into the computer, the following results were produced:

$$R = .208 \qquad R\text{-square} = .043$$
$$\text{Slope (Predictor)} = .101 \qquad \text{Constant (Y-intercept)} = 1.327$$

The following information can be plugged into the regression equation:

$$Y = .101 (30) + 1.327 = 4.357$$

The slope was equal to .101, and that was multiplied by the average number of referrals over the past nine-month period (30). The Y-intercept of 1.327 was added to the product, leading to a sum of 4.357. With this being rounded out to 4, you forecasted that during the next month, the facility could anticipate four admissions that would result given the predictor variable and the average number of referrals. The R = .208 is the association between the two variables. The R-square indicates the amount of total variation that can be accounted for by the equation. For example, if R = 1.00, R-square would be 1.00, accounting for all the variation. If R = .50, R-square would be equal to 0.25, accounting for only 25% of the variation. This is an important indicator, in which the greater levels of variation that are accounted for lead to more confidence in the results obtained. In this example, the R-square is not inspiring.

Dummy variable regression analysis

Another type of regression analysis is *dummy variable regression analysis*. Using this technique involves using *dummy variables*, which are binary variables, either 0 or 1, with 0 usually standing for the absence of something and 1 standing for the presence of something. The concept of dummy variable regression analysis is the same as that for bivariate regression analysis. The only difference is that the predictor variable has a binary categorization. Through the use of the dummy variable associated with an independent variable, a healthcare administrator can conduct regression analysis to help forecast phenomena that can possibly aid in his or her managerial decisions.

For example, say you are interested in determining how nursing staffing affects the number of falls that occur within a given 24-hour period. You examine data from the past 30 days. If the staffing met or exceeded the guidelines established by the U.S. Department of Health and Human Services, you entered the dummy variable 1 for that day. You also entered the number of falls that occurred during that day. If the staffing did not meet the recommended guidelines that were established, you entered a 0 as well as the respective number of falls, if any, that occurred during that 24-hour period. After entering the data into the computer, you obtained the following results:

$$R = .677 \qquad R\text{-Square} = .458$$
$$\text{Slope (predictor)} = -1.550 \qquad \text{Constant (Y-intercept)} = 2.00$$

$$Y' = -1.550 (1) + 2.00 = 0.45$$
or
$$Y' = -1.550 (0) + 2.00 = 2.00$$

Over the next 10 days, you notice that adequate staffing was found for each of those days. Given the dummy variables used as predictor variables, you noticed that during the next 10 days during which adequate staffing was found, the forecasted likelihood of falls on those days was statistically less than one fall per day. However, on day 11, when staffing was under the recommended level, the forecasted number of falls for that 24-hour period was two. Furthermore, the R = 0.677 indicates that there was a strong relationship between staffing and falls. Also, when the R-square is evaluated in relation to the higher correlation between the variables, a much larger amount of the total variation, R-square = 0.458, is accounted for in this example than in the previous example.

John Stuart Mill: The Logic Behind Causal Understanding

The prominent utilitarian philosopher John Stuart Mill developed a system of logic that is still used today. His two major methods for making logical comparisons are called the *method of agreement* and

CHAPTER 18

the *method of difference*. These approaches seek to give a causal explanation by examining the regularities within a particular context under examination (Neuman, 2000). By examining points of agreement and areas of differences, healthcare professionals can employ a logical method of reasoning for understanding the causative nature behind a given event or phenomenon. Although these are not often mentioned within healthcare administration circles as important techniques to use for data evaluation, they can be productive.

The method of agreement

In the method of agreement, the healthcare administrator would focus his or her attention on what is common across a number of cases. The cases can be individuals, groups, healthcare institutions, large corporations, or societies as a whole. For example, say that as a consultant for a large long-term care corporation, you have been called in to evaluate why resident-to-resident abuse is much higher in four of your facilities compared to the other facilities that all have much lower levels of resident-to-resident abuse. In doing this comparative analysis, you examine a number of variables, such as levels of dementia, activities offered, levels of medication use, and staff training. Each of the letters in the following table stands for a particular coded feature that you examine to help determine some type of causal analysis.

You examine each nursing facility as a separate case and then compare the cases to each other, in turn examining each case for similarities that may indicate a causal answer for the higher rates of resident-to-resident altercations. After examining the data, you notice two similarities among all four nursing facilities: All four had high rates (more than 80%) of residents with dementia, and all four had staff members who had little, if any, training in behavioral management. These are denoted by the variables A and B. The letters that I used to stand for variables are just random. However, in reality, you often would use letters or some type of notation for a variable as a shorthand way to analyze the data.

Method of Agreement

Case 1	Case 2	Case 3	Case 4
a	a	a	a
b	b	b	b
c	c	d	e
f	f	g	h
i	j	k	k
l	m	l	n
o	o	p	q

THE TIME VALUE OF MONEY AND FORECASTING

The preceding example demonstrates four cases that share two similar features that may be causative in the resident-to-resident abuse you are evaluating. After this, however, each of the four facilities differs markedly in the other variables. From this data, you can determine that in all four facilities that experienced higher rates of resident-to-resident abuse, they also shared (or had in agreement) higher levels of residents with dementia and staff members who were poorly trained in behavioral management.

The method of difference

In some examples, the cases may be in agreement in some areas but may fail to have the same results. For example, what happens when, in the preceding example, some of the cases that shared similar variables did not experience the same high rates of resident-to-resident abuse? In this case, the method of difference can deal with those subtle nuances that bring about differences that are not caught by the method of agreement.

The method of difference gives the researcher a stronger ability to understand the logic of causal analysis. It is more or less a "double application" of the method of agreement, in which you first examine cases that share a similarity in many areas, while at the same time being attentive to the differences that are found in crucial areas (Neuman, 2000). By examining those cases that share many features and do not end up with the same results, while paying close attention to some of the subtle discrepancies that may have caused these differences to transpire, you can logically extrapolate, even with greater certainty than in the method of agreement, the causal analysis for a particular phenomenon. Again, the following example will help to demonstrate this technique:

Method of Difference

Case 1	Case 2	Case 5	Case 6
a	a	x	a
b	b	z	q
c	c	d	c
f	f	f	f
i	j	k	k
l	m	l	n
o	o	o	q

Finance, Budgeting & Quantitative Analysis: A Primer for Nursing Home Administrators

CHAPTER 18

In this example, the letter (a) stands for high levels of dementia in the population and (b) stands for low levels of behavioral training among the staff. As you look through the matrix, you'll notice that cases 1 and 2 (facilities within the corporation that have higher levels of resident-to-resident abuse) and cases 5 and 6 (facilities in the corporation that have much lower levels of resident-to-resident abuse) share many of the same variables. In fact, in the fourth line down, each case shares that same variable (f), despite dramatically different outcomes related to resident abuse.

However, the critical difference that appears to explain the cause of why cases 1 and 2 had higher rates of resident-to-resident abuse than cases 5 and 6, which failed to have these same high rates, is found in the second line of the table. It appears that in cases 5 and 6, two different types of behavioral management techniques were used consistently by all staff members, who had extensive training in their application. As such, it appears that the critical factor that is causing the difference between the facilities is not so much the level of dementia as the training of the staff.

The method of difference is slightly more complicated than the method of agreement, but it offers more powerful logic in causal analysis. By examining both areas of agreement as well as differences, one is able to logically determine cause with greater certainty than one could do using just the method of agreement.

THE TIME VALUE OF MONEY AND FORECASTING

FIGURE 18.6
PRESENT VALUE OF $1

$$\$1 = (1+r)^{-n}$$

r = discount rate   n = number of periods until payment

Years	1.00%	2.00%	3.00%	4.00%	5.00%	6.00%	7.00%	8.00%	9.00%	10.00%	11.00%	12.00%	13.00%	14.00%	15.00%
1	$0.99010	$0.98039	$0.97087	$0.96154	$0.95238	$0.94340	$0.93458	$0.92593	$0.91743	$0.90909	$0.90090	$0.89286	$0.88496	$0.87719	$0.86957
2	$0.98030	$0.96117	$0.94260	$0.92456	$0.90703	$0.89000	$0.87344	$0.85734	$0.84168	$0.82645	$0.81162	$0.79719	$0.78315	$0.76947	$0.75614
3	$0.97059	$0.94232	$0.91514	$0.88900	$0.86384	$0.83962	$0.81630	$0.79383	$0.77218	$0.75132	$0.73119	$0.71178	$0.69305	$0.67497	$0.65752
4	$0.96098	$0.92385	$0.88849	$0.85480	$0.82270	$0.79209	$0.76290	$0.73503	$0.70843	$0.68301	$0.65873	$0.63552	$0.61332	$0.59208	$0.57175
5	$0.95147	$0.90573	$0.86261	$0.82193	$0.78353	$0.74726	$0.71299	$0.68058	$0.64993	$0.62092	$0.59345	$0.56743	$0.54276	$0.51937	$0.49718
6	$0.94205	$0.88797	$0.83748	$0.79032	$0.74622	$0.70496	$0.66634	$0.63017	$0.59627	$0.56447	$0.53464	$0.50663	$0.48032	$0.45559	$0.43233
7	$0.93272	$0.87056	$0.81309	$0.75992	$0.71068	$0.66506	$0.62275	$0.58349	$0.54703	$0.51316	$0.48166	$0.45235	$0.42506	$0.39964	$0.37594
8	$0.92348	$0.85349	$0.78941	$0.73069	$0.67684	$0.62741	$0.58201	$0.54027	$0.50187	$0.46651	$0.43393	$0.40388	$0.37616	$0.35056	$0.32690
9	$0.91434	$0.83676	$0.76642	$0.70259	$0.64461	$0.59190	$0.54393	$0.50025	$0.46043	$0.42410	$0.39093	$0.36061	$0.33289	$0.30751	$0.28426
10	$0.90529	$0.82035	$0.74409	$0.67556	$0.61391	$0.55840	$0.50835	$0.46319	$0.42241	$0.38554	$0.35218	$0.32197	$0.29459	$0.26974	$0.24719
11	$0.89632	$0.80426	$0.72242	$0.64958	$0.58468	$0.52679	$0.47509	$0.42888	$0.38753	$0.35049	$0.31728	$0.28748	$0.26070	$0.23662	$0.21494
12	$0.88745	$0.78849	$0.70138	$0.62460	$0.55684	$0.49697	$0.44401	$0.39711	$0.35554	$0.31863	$0.28584	$0.25668	$0.23071	$0.20756	$0.18691
13	$0.87866	$0.77303	$0.68095	$0.60057	$0.53032	$0.46884	$0.41496	$0.36770	$0.32618	$0.28966	$0.25751	$0.22917	$0.20417	$0.18207	$0.16253
14	$0.86996	$0.75788	$0.66112	$0.57748	$0.50507	$0.44230	$0.38782	$0.34046	$0.29925	$0.26333	$0.23200	$0.20462	$0.18068	$0.15971	$0.14133
15	$0.86135	$0.74301	$0.64186	$0.55527	$0.48102	$0.41727	$0.36245	$0.31524	$0.27454	$0.23939	$0.20900	$0.18270	$0.15989	$0.14010	$0.12289
16	$0.85282	$0.72845	$0.62317	$0.53391	$0.45811	$0.39365	$0.33874	$0.29189	$0.25187	$0.21763	$0.18829	$0.16312	$0.14150	$0.12289	$0.10687
17	$0.84438	$0.71416	$0.60502	$0.51337	$0.43630	$0.37136	$0.31657	$0.27027	$0.23107	$0.19785	$0.16963	$0.14564	$0.12522	$0.10780	$0.09293
18	$0.83602	$0.70016	$0.58740	$0.49363	$0.41552	$0.35034	$0.29586	$0.25025	$0.21199	$0.17986	$0.15282	$0.13004	$0.11081	$0.09456	$0.08081
19	$0.82774	$0.68643	$0.57029	$0.47464	$0.39573	$0.33051	$0.27651	$0.23171	$0.19449	$0.16351	$0.13768	$0.11611	$0.09806	$0.08295	$0.07027
20	$0.81954	$0.67297	$0.55368	$0.45639	$0.37689	$0.31181	$0.25842	$0.21455	$0.17843	$0.14864	$0.12403	$0.10367	$0.08678	$0.07276	$0.06110
21	$0.81143	$0.65978	$0.53755	$0.43883	$0.35894	$0.29416	$0.24151	$0.19866	$0.16370	$0.13513	$0.11174	$0.09256	$0.07680	$0.06383	$0.05313
22	$0.80340	$0.64684	$0.52189	$0.42196	$0.34185	$0.27751	$0.22571	$0.18394	$0.15018	$0.12285	$0.10067	$0.08264	$0.06796	$0.05599	$0.04620
23	$0.79544	$0.63416	$0.50669	$0.40573	$0.32557	$0.26180	$0.21095	$0.17032	$0.13778	$0.11168	$0.09069	$0.07379	$0.06014	$0.04911	$0.04017
24	$0.78757	$0.62172	$0.49193	$0.39012	$0.31007	$0.24698	$0.19715	$0.15770	$0.12641	$0.10153	$0.08171	$0.06588	$0.05323	$0.04308	$0.03493
25	$0.77977	$0.60953	$0.47761	$0.37512	$0.29530	$0.23300	$0.18425	$0.14602	$0.11597	$0.09230	$0.07361	$0.05882	$0.04710	$0.03779	$0.03038

CHAPTER 18

FIGURE 18.7
FUTURE VALUE OF $1

Period	1%	2%	3%	4%	5%	6%	7%	8%	9%	10%
1	1.01000	1.02000	1.03000	1.04000	1.05000	1.06000	1.07000	1.08000	1.09000	1.10000
2	1.02010	1.04040	1.06090	1.08160	1.10250	1.12360	1.14490	1.16640	1.18810	1.21000
3	1.03030	1.06121	1.09273	1.12486	1.15763	1.19102	1.22504	1.25971	1.29503	1.33100
4	1.04060	1.08243	1.12551	1.16986	1.21551	1.26248	1.31080	1.36049	1.41158	1.46410
5	1.05101	1.10408	1.15927	1.21665	1.27628	1.33823	1.40255	1.46933	1.53862	1.61051
6	1.06152	1.12616	1.19405	1.26532	1.34010	1.41852	1.50073	1.58687	1.67710	1.77156
7	1.07214	1.14869	1.22987	1.31593	1.40710	1.50363	1.60578	1.71382	1.82804	1.94872
8	1.08286	1.17166	1.26677	1.36857	1.47746	1.59385	1.71819	1.85093	1.99256	2.14359
9	1.09369	1.19509	1.30477	1.42331	1.55133	1.68948	1.83846	1.99900	2.17189	2.35795
10	1.10462	1.21899	1.34392	1.48024	1.62889	1.79085	1.96715	2.15892	2.36736	2.59374
11	1.11567	1.24337	1.38423	1.53945	1.71034	1.89830	2.10485	2.33164	2.58043	2.85312
12	1.12683	1.26824	1.42576	1.60103	1.79586	2.01220	2.25219	2.51817	2.81266	3.13843
13	1.13809	1.29361	1.46853	1.66507	1.88565	2.13293	2.40985	2.71962	3.06580	3.45227
14	1.14947	1.31948	1.51259	1.73168	1.97993	2.26090	2.57853	2.93719	3.34173	3.79750
15	1.16097	1.34587	1.55797	1.80094	2.07893	2.39656	2.75903	3.17217	3.64248	4.17725
16	1.17258	1.37279	1.60471	1.87298	2.18287	2.54035	2.95216	3.42594	3.97031	4.59497
17	1.18430	1.40024	1.65285	1.94790	2.29202	2.69277	3.15882	3.70002	4.32763	5.05447
18	1.19615	1.42825	1.70243	2.02582	2.40662	2.85434	3.37993	3.99602	4.71712	5.55992
19	1.20811	1.45681	1.75351	2.10685	2.52695	3.02560	3.61653	4.31570	5.14166	6.11591
20	1.22019	1.48595	1.80611	2.19112	2.65330	3.20714	3.86968	4.66096	5.60441	6.72750
21	1.23239	1.51567	1.86029	2.27877	2.78596	3.39956	4.14056	5.03383	6.10881	7.40025
22	1.24472	1.54598	1.91610	2.36992	2.92526	3.60354	4.43040	5.43654	6.65860	8.14027
23	1.25716	1.57690	1.97359	2.46472	3.07152	3.81975	4.74053	5.87146	7.25787	8.95430
24	1.26973	1.60844	2.03279	2.56330	3.22510	4.04893	5.07237	6.34118	7.91108	9.84973
25	1.28243	1.64061	2.09378	2.66584	3.38635	4.29187	5.42743	6.84848	8.62308	10.83471
26	1.29526	1.67342	2.15659	2.77247	3.55567	4.54938	5.80735	7.39635	9.39916	11.91818
27	1.30821	1.70689	2.22129	2.88337	3.73346	4.82235	6.21387	7.98806	10.24508	13.10999
28	1.32129	1.74102	2.28793	2.99870	3.92013	5.11169	6.64884	8.62711	11.16714	14.42099
29	1.33450	1.77584	2.35657	3.11865	4.11614	5.41839	7.11426	9.31727	12.17218	15.86309
30	1.34785	1.81136	2.42726	3.24340	4.32194	5.74349	7.61226	10.06266	13.26768	17.44940
31	1.36133	1.84759	2.50008	3.37313	4.53804	6.08810	8.14511	10.86767	14.46177	19.19434
32	1.37494	1.88454	2.57508	3.50806	4.76494	6.45339	8.71527	11.73708	15.76333	21.11378
33	1.38869	1.92223	2.65234	3.64838	5.00319	6.84059	9.32534	12.67605	17.18203	23.22515
34	1.40258	1.96068	2.73191	3.79432	5.25335	7.25103	9.97811	13.69013	18.72841	25.54767
35	1.41660	1.99989	2.81386	3.94609	5.51602	7.68609	10.67658	14.78534	20.41397	28.10244
36	1.43077	2.03989	2.89828	4.10393	5.79182	8.14725	11.42394	15.96817	22.25123	30.91268
37	1.44508	2.08069	2.98523	4.26809	6.08141	8.63609	12.22362	17.24563	24.25384	34.00395
38	1.45953	2.12230	3.07478	4.43881	6.38548	9.15425	13.07927	18.62528	26.43668	37.40434
39	1.47412	2.16474	3.16703	4.61637	6.70475	9.70351	13.99482	20.11530	28.81598	41.14478
40	1.48886	2.20804	3.26204	4.80102	7.03999	10.28572	14.97446	21.72452	31.40942	45.25926

THE TIME VALUE OF MONEY AND FORECASTING

FIGURE 18.7
FUTURE VALUE OF $1 (CONT.)

12%	14%	15%	16%	18%	20%	24%	28%	32%	36%
1.12000	1.14000	1.15000	1.16000	1.18000	1.20000	1.24000	1.28000	1.32000	1.36000
1.25440	1.29960	1.32250	1.34560	1.39240	1.44000	1.53760	1.63840	1.74240	1.84960
1.40493	1.48154	1.52088	1.56090	1.64303	1.72800	1.90662	2.09715	2.29997	2.51546
1.57352	1.68896	1.74901	1.81064	1.93878	2.07360	2.36421	2.68435	3.03596	3.42102
1.76234	1.92541	2.01136	2.10034	2.28776	2.48832	2.93163	3.43597	4.00746	4.65259
1.97382	2.19497	2.31306	2.43640	2.69955	2.98598	3.63522	4.39805	5.28985	6.32752
2.21068	2.50227	2.66002	2.82622	3.18547	3.58318	4.50767	5.62950	6.98261	8.60543
2.47596	2.85259	3.05902	3.27841	3.75886	4.29982	5.58951	7.20576	9.21704	11.70338
2.77308	3.25195	3.51788	3.80296	4.43545	5.15978	6.93099	9.22337	12.16649	15.91660
3.10585	3.70722	4.04556	4.41144	5.23384	6.19174	8.59443	11.80592	16.05977	21.64657
3.47855	4.22623	4.65239	5.11726	6.17593	7.43008	10.65709	15.11157	21.19890	29.43933
3.89598	4.81790	5.35025	5.93603	7.28759	8.91610	13.21479	19.34281	27.98254	40.03750
4.36349	5.49241	6.15279	6.88579	8.59936	10.69932	16.38634	24.75880	36.93696	54.45099
4.88711	6.26135	7.07571	7.98752	10.14724	12.83918	20.31906	31.69127	48.75678	74.05335
5.47357	7.13794	8.13706	9.26552	11.97375	15.40702	25.19563	40.56482	64.35895	100.713
6.13039	8.13725	9.35762	10.74800	14.12902	18.48843	31.24259	51.92297	84.95382	136.969
6.86604	9.27646	10.76126	12.46768	16.67225	22.18611	38.74081	66.46140	112.139	186.278
7.68997	10.57517	12.37545	14.46251	19.67325	26.62333	48.03860	85.07059	148.024	253.338
8.61276	12.05569	14.23177	16.77652	23.21444	31.94800	59.56786	108.890	195.391	344.540
9.64629	13.74349	16.36654	19.46076	27.39303	38.33760	73.86415	139.380	257.916	468.574
10.80385	15.66758	18.82152	22.57448	32.32378	46.00512	91.59155	178.406	340.449	637.261
12.10031	17.86104	21.64475	26.18640	38.14206	55.20614	113.574	228.360	449.393	866.674
13.55235	20.36158	24.89146	30.37622	45.00763	66.24737	140.831	292.300	593.199	1178.677
15.17863	23.21221	28.62518	35.23642	53.10901	79.49685	174.631	374.144	783.023	1603.001
17.00006	26.46192	32.91895	40.87424	62.66863	95.39622	216.542	478.905	1033.590	2180.081
19.04007	30.16658	37.85680	47.41412	73.94898	114.475	268.512	612.998	1364.339	2964.911
21.32488	34.38991	43.53531	55.00038	87.25980	137.371	332.955	784.638	1800.927	4032.279
23.88387	39.20449	50.06561	63.80044	102.967	164.845	412.864	1004.336	2377.224	5483.899
26.74993	44.69312	57.57545	74.00851	121.501	197.814	511.952	1285.550	3137.935	7458.102
29.95992	50.95016	66.21177	85.84988	143.371	237.376	634.820	1645.505	4142.075	10143.019
33.55511	58.08318	76.14354	99.58586	169.177	284.852	787.177	2106.246	5467.539	13794.506
37.58173	66.21483	87.56507	115.520	199.629	341.822	976.099	2695.995	7217.151	18760.528
42.09153	75.48490	100.700	134.003	235.563	410.186	1210.363	3450.873	9526.639	25514.319
47.14252	86.05279	115.805	155.443	277.964	492.224	1500.850	4417.118	12575.164	34699.473
52.79962	98.10018	133.176	180.314	327.997	590.668	1861.054	5653.911	16599.217	47191.284
59.13557	111.834	153.152	209.164	387.037	708.802	2307.707	7237.006	21910.966	64180.146
66.23184	127.491	176.125	242.631	456.703	850.562	2861.557	9263.367	28922.475	87284.999
74.17966	145.340	202.543	281.452	538.910	1020.675	3548.330	11857.110	38177.667	118707.598
83.08122	165.687	232.925	326.484	635.914	1224.810	4399.930	15177.101	50394.520	161442.334
93.05097	188.884	267.864	378.721	750.378	1469.772	5455.913	19426.689	66520.767	219561.574

Note: To view the full version of this figure, please refer to the downloadable materials that accompany this book.

19 Planning Through the Use of Networks

Network analysis is a quantitative technique used for project planning. This type of analysis was highly popular at one time and is still used in various forms to analyze important managerial decisions for major projects. In other words, it is not a technique that is used for the types of common, day-to-day problems encountered by healthcare administrators. Nonetheless, it is important to understand the concept and how it can relate to decision-making in the healthcare arena.

Program Evaluation Review Technique

Probably the most common form of network analysis is the Program Evaluation Review Technique (PERT). One of the major strengths of this type of analysis is that it helps to organize, structure, and set timetables for planning and project development.

Determining an estimated time of completion for projects through structuring the organization of the steps involved is very important. It helps to provide timelines for your project management by estimated time values.

In developing a network analysis using PERT, you must first establish the goals of the program and when the program must be complete. For example, say that while planning for your next year's budget, you must incorporate a new project: a new Alzheimer's unit. It is August, and the new unit is scheduled to open the following February. You need to finalize your budget by October. That means you have a timeline of five months for the project to be completed. The new wing will be placed in an existing part of the facility and will have 24 beds. Your first step is to determine the order in which the project should be completed (see the figure below).

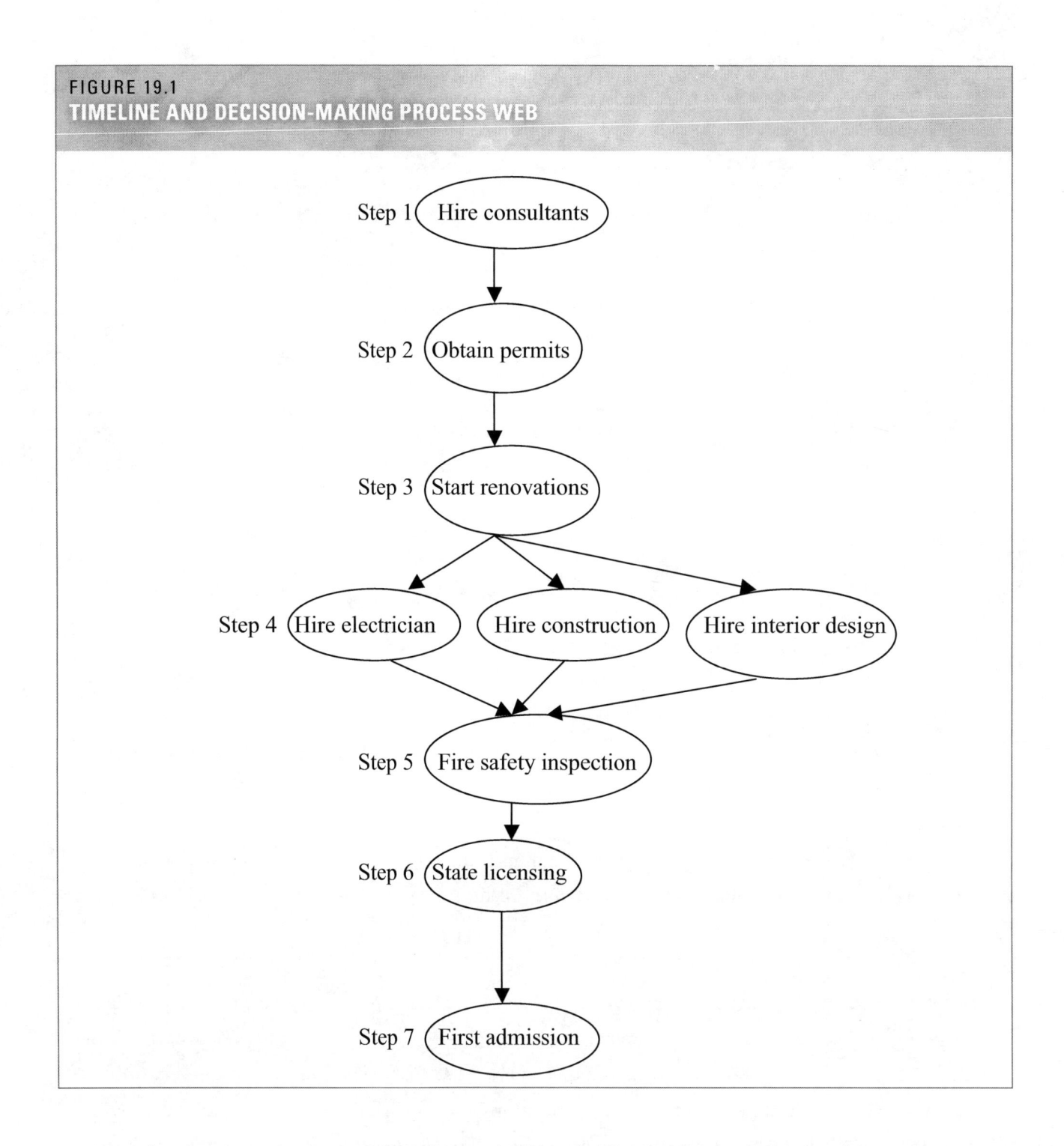

FIGURE 19.1
TIMELINE AND DECISION-MAKING PROCESS WEB

- Step 1: Hire consultants
- Step 2: Obtain permits
- Step 3: Start renovations
- Step 4: Hire electrician / Hire construction / Hire interior design
- Step 5: Fire safety inspection
- Step 6: State licensing
- Step 7: First admission

Note that the arrows in the preceding diagram indicate the direction of the decision-making process. In this example, the steps are simplistic; in real-world projects, however, such a diagram would likely include several arrows moving in many different directions.

PLANNING THROUGH THE USE OF NETWORKS

After you have determined the order in which the tasks need to be accomplished, you must estimate how long each task will take to be completed. PERT traditionally places three estimates on each line for each task: the least amount of time the task is likely to take, your estimate for the amount of time the task is likely to take, and the most amount of time the task is likely to take. For example, the timeline from the time of hiring a consultant to the time the permits will be issued may be as follows:

- The least amount of time this will take is two weeks

- Most likely, this will take four weeks

- The most amount of time this will take is six weeks

After you've made these estimations, you can determine the estimated time periods, using the following formula:

$$\text{Estimated time period or (te)} = \frac{le + 4m + lo}{6}$$

Where:

- te = expected amount of time

- le = least amount of time

- m = most likely amount of time

- lo = longest time of time

Therefore, the expected amount of time for the project to be completed is as follows:

$$\text{Estimated time period or (te)} = \frac{2 + 4(4) + 6}{6} = 4$$

Finance, Budgeting & Quantitative Analysis: A Primer for Nursing Home Administrators

CHAPTER 19

It is important to realize that the expected time that is calculated is only as good as your estimates of least amount of time, most likely amount of time, and longest amount of time. Although the formula can help you to determine the expected amount of time this task will take, the data you input into the formula is, for the most part, subjective.

Often, a project involves many paths. Because networks often have many tasks that lead to a common end, PERT analysis frequently speaks about the critical path, which is the longest path or time estimate for the completion of a particular stage of a project. The figure below demonstrates this.

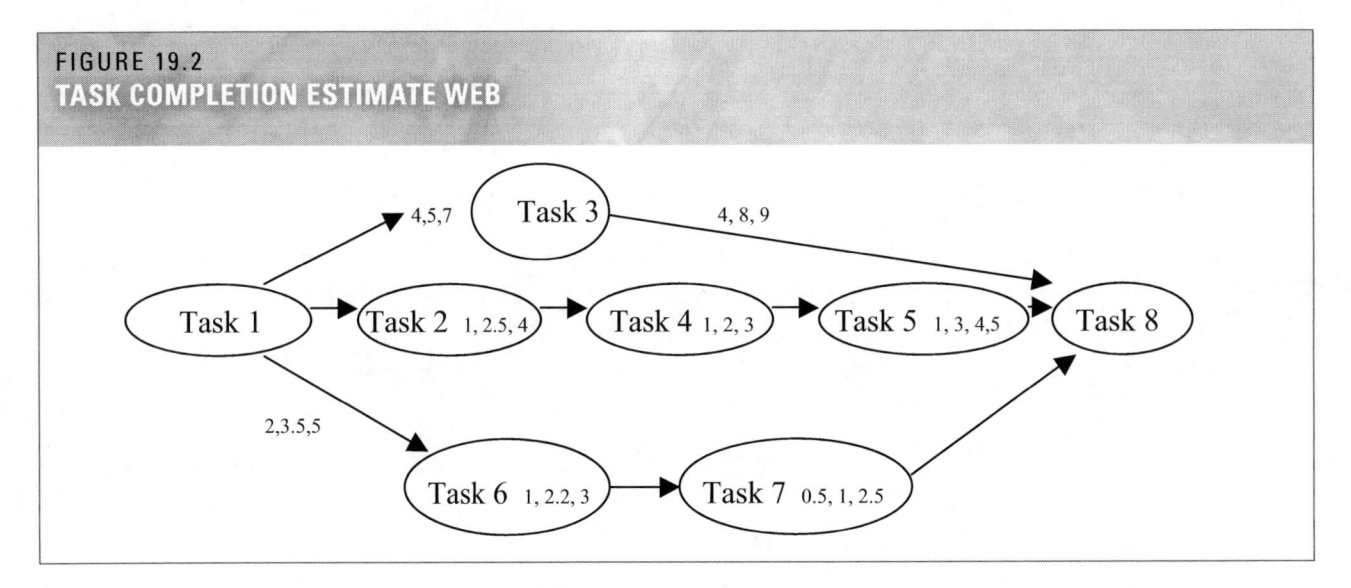

FIGURE 19.2
TASK COMPLETION ESTIMATE WEB

```
                    4,5,7    Task 3    4, 8, 9
                   ↗                            ↘
    Task 1 → Task 2  1, 2.5, 4 → Task 4  1, 2, 3 → Task 5  1, 3, 4,5 → Task 8
         ↘                                                              ↗
          2,3.5,5
                   Task 6  1, 2.2, 3 → Task 7  0.5, 1, 2.5
```

Notice that each task has next to it three numbers which denote the least expected amount of time, the most likely amount of time, and the longest anticipated amount of time. Also notice in the top path that the number of months it will take to complete this project is 5 + 8 = 13 months. In the middle path, going from task 1 to 2, 2 to 4, 4 to 5, and 5 to 8, it will take 3 + 2.5 + 2 + 3 = 10.5 months. Finally, the third path, going from task 1 to 6, 6 to 7, and 7 to 8, will take 3.5 + 2.2 + 1 = 6.7 months. Therefore, to finish the project in the least amount of time, you would follow the last path.

PERT analysis has other features, but I feel its best attribute is that it provides a visual model for your planning. In doing so, it qualitatively places organizational time estimates on what needs to be done, along with when it needs to be done. Because planning and finance are strongly linked, this helps you to monitor your control of the time and task schedule, which, if not monitored closely, can lead to unneeded expenditures due to poor time management.

PLANNING THROUGH THE USE OF NETWORKS

Decision-Making in Long-Term Care

The level of information that you have in order to make decisions in healthcare settings often differs dramatically. Decisions are often incumbent on the level of information that is available to the decision-makers. Administrators face these issues daily when making decisions. Therefore, it is important for administrators to realize that decision-making is not a one-dimensional process. Although individuals often think of decision-making as "taking a stand" and "being decisive," the complexity of decisions is predicated on more than these trite explanations; the type and amount of information that lends itself to administrators and the administrative staff has to also be taken into consideration.

For example, in understanding the complexity of your decisions, you have to evaluate whether you are dealing with a programmed or a nonprogrammed decision. These two distinctions are common in long-term care management.

Programmed and Nonprogrammed Decisions

Programmed decisions occur frequently. Because they occur frequently, there are often well-developed types of procedures and rules that guide decisions in these areas. They are also often habitual patterns of decisions that we have engaged in frequently. Take, for example, the frequent issue of dealing with disciplinary actions regarding employee absenteeism or tardiness. Because this is a recurrent issue, decision rules in this area are not only explicitly stated but also implicitly determined. Programmed decisions often are made when administrators must deal with routine survey issues. But one of the most common programmed decisions that many administrators deal with is examining their costs in relation to their budget and their per patient days to ensure that costs do not exceed these areas; if they do, administrators need to make an adjustment in their daily workforce, which is another programmed decision.

Conversely, nonprogrammed decisions are encountered in situations that occur less frequently, and therefore they are more unusual. Often, there fails to be well-established decision rules for dealing with these issues, and because of their less frequent occurrence, administrators often face greater levels of ambiguity in addressing these concerns. Because of the unique situations that are frequently part of nonprogrammed decisions, the lack of routine that is part of programmed decision-making leads to a comfort zone that is much less secure for many administrators. These types of decisions often provoke some level of anxiety and trepidation.

Finance, Budgeting & Quantitative Analysis: A Primer for Nursing Home Administrators

CHAPTER 19

Examples of problems that require nonprogrammed decisions include those that deal with abuse, fires and evacuation, or being informed that there needs to be an immediate abatement to an immediate jeopardy citation. Another example is the decision of whether to establish a bariatric unit. Even the best administrators cannot anticipate every contingency, and although you may have layers of policies that in some way address many of the issues regarding the benefits and limitations of establishing a bariatric unit in your facility, such a situation will supersede simulation and paper policies. Furthermore, venturing into a new area that may incur costs but that also may raise considerable revenue always comes with a level of risk.

Some problems—specifically, those that deal with interfacility differences—may require both programmed and nonprogrammed decisions. For example, say that facility A deals with a high level of acuity as it relates to issues of bariatric residents. Emergent issues related to bariatric residents may be routine and part of daily programmed decision-making strategies in this facility. However, facility B has a lower acuity and may not deal with the needs of bariatric residents as routinely as facility A does. Therefore, if a bariatric resident at facility B becomes severely compromised, the decision rules may be more ambiguous because this facility has not dealt frequently with this type of issue.

So, what is a programmed decision in one facility may actually be a nonprogrammed decision in another. Administrators have to be aware of common facility-to-facility programmed decisions as well as the variances among facilities that lead to nonprogrammed decisions.

Conditions of Certainty, Uncertainty, and Risk

Healthcare decisions, regardless of whether they are programmed or nonprogrammed, can also exist under conditions of certainty, uncertainty, and risk. In some cases, the decisions that are made exist under conditions of certainty, in which the outcomes and alternatives to particular outcomes are known. In this situation, administrators have a clear understanding of the alternatives and how each alternative will impact the healthcare facility. If a facility has, for example, $30,000 to spend for capital improvement and two areas need improvement, the kitchen and physical therapy, what is spent on the kitchen becomes an opportunity cost to physical therapy. If $20,000 is spent on the kitchen, it is clear that only $10,000 exists for physical therapy enhancement.

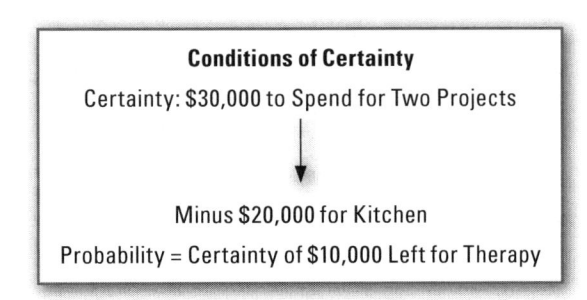

PLANNING THROUGH THE USE OF NETWORKS

Conditions of Certainty

Certainty: $30,000 to Spend for Two Projects

↓

Minus $20,000 for Kitchen

Probability = Certainty of $10,000 Left for Therapy

With conditions of uncertainty, there is not enough information to make a clear decision and be able to understand how making a decision will influence alternative outcomes. Under these circumstances, some individuals will guess at what they "think" is the right decision. Administrators often like to use the "based on my years of experience" argument to justify their decisions when they lack information. However, when you're dealing with human lives, the most prudent means are often to seek more information so that you can act more judiciously.

For example, say you have to decide whether to promote your nursing home to help increase your census, but you have no existing information on which to base that decision.

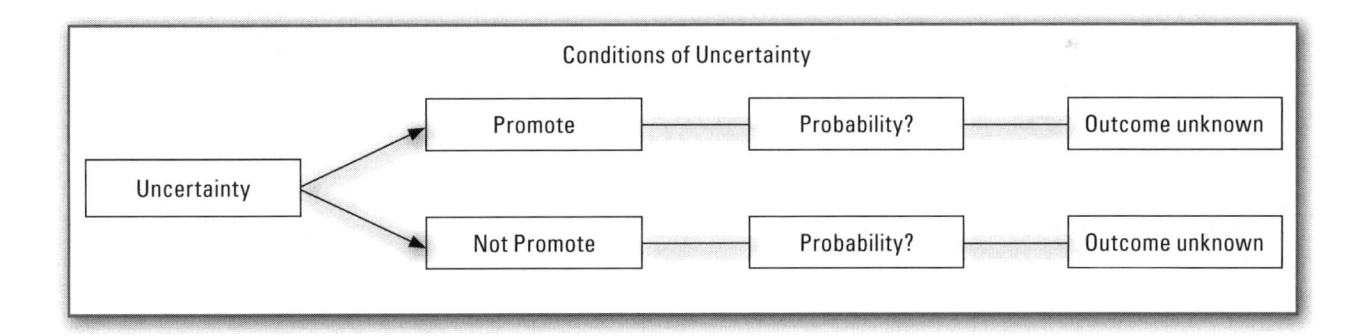

Conditions of Uncertainty

Uncertainty → Promote → Probability? → Outcome unknown

Uncertainty → Not Promote → Probability? → Outcome unknown

Probably the most difficult decisions administrators face are those that incur some probability of risk, where they are unable to know with certainty what outcome given actions will have after decisions are made. Many financial and planning decisions fall under this category. Under these conditions of risk, there is often enough information available to the administrator to make informed decisions based on a level of probability. However, just because you make a decision based on an 80% probability that, for example, the payback period for purchasing a piece of equipment will be six months or less or that there is an 80% probability that instituting a wage increase will reduce nursing turnover by 50% does not mean that this will always be the case.

CHAPTER 19

In addition, it is common to make decisions based on probability but to delude ourselves into thinking that the probability will become the actual occurrence. Psychologically, this helps us feel better about decisions that often incur risk. However, just because the probability of, for example, a tossed penny landing heads or tails is 50% and that it has turned up heads on the first toss does not mean the probability that it will land tails on the second toss increases. The probability still remains at 50%.

To demonstrate the condition of risk, say you want to add an Alzheimer's unit to your facility, but you are unsure of the size or whether, regardless of size, adding the unit would be more profitable than just adding a similar number of skilled beds.

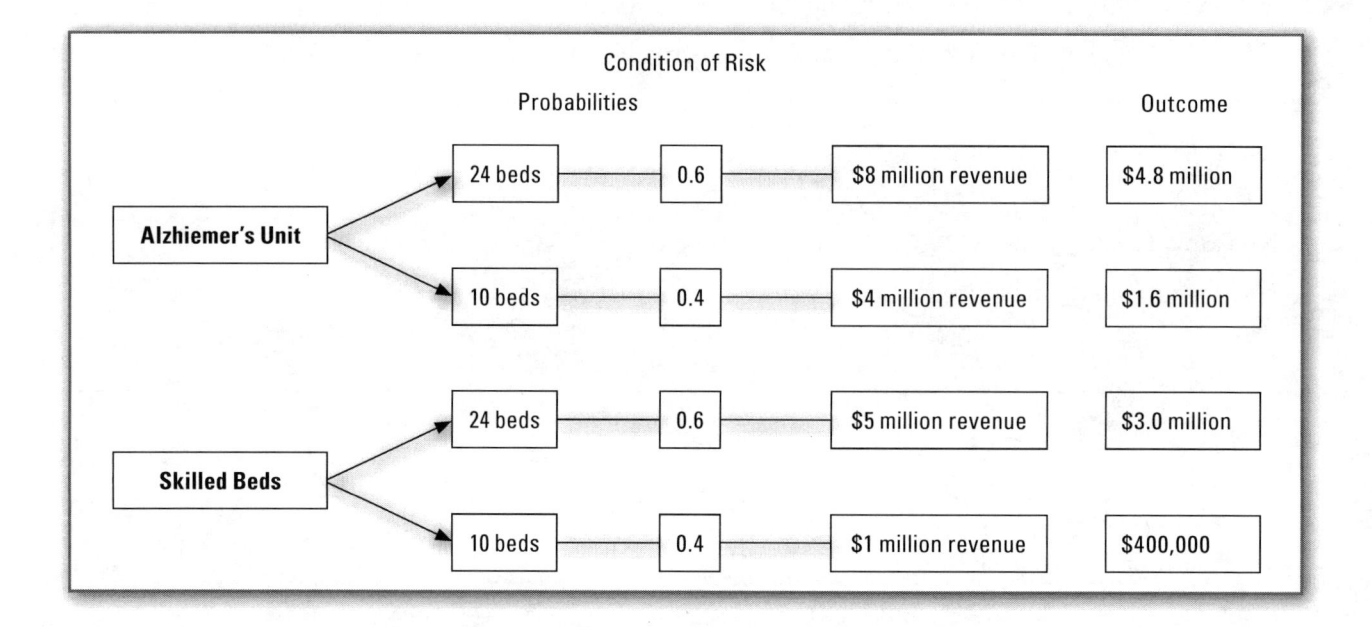

Condition of Risk

Option	Beds	Probability	Revenue	Outcome
Alzhiemer's Unit	24 beds	0.6	$8 million revenue	$4.8 million
Alzhiemer's Unit	10 beds	0.4	$4 million revenue	$1.6 million
Skilled Beds	24 beds	0.6	$5 million revenue	$3.0 million
Skilled Beds	10 beds	0.4	$1 million revenue	$400,000

Given these probabilities, if known, multiplied by the expected revenue, we get a particular outcome against which we can gauge our decision-making. However, here is the risk. Often, the probability is not an objective probability but rather a subjective probability. If you can ascertain an objective probability, that helps to reduce the risk. However, because many probabilities are estimated guesses, that can increase the risk involved in decision-making.

At first blush, it appears in the preceding example that the 24-bed Alzheimer's unit may be the best investment and that even when it is averaged over the 24 beds, roughly $200,000 in revenue is realized for each bed, which is more than the other three alternatives. But this does not capture the full risk. To

PLANNING THROUGH THE USE OF NETWORKS

provide a better picture of this issue, it may be helpful to have anticipated costs and the probability for the anticipated costs as it relates to the respective bed size. We can do this via a simple decision-tree analysis.

For many, decision-making appears to be a clear and easy process. However, as discussed in the preceding paragraphs, decisions hold a level of complexity that is often not recognized. Long-term care administrators face many different types of decisions, and it is important for them to understand that decision-making is more than just an arbitrary and capricious endeavor. Yet, understanding the decision-making process, the types of decisions you'll need to make, and the challenges you'll face in dealing with this important task will help you to deal with the anxiety that is part of decision-making. Therefore, decision-making is a skill that you can improve by being cognizant of the types of decisions you are presented with, the common problems that exist in making decisions, and the ability to recognize your strengths and weaknesses in this area.

20 Basic Economic Principles

The economic institution in centered on the economic resources it uses in the production of goods and services. Healthcare is an important resource, and the healthcare administrator should have some understanding of basic economic principles. Consider the following:

- Healthcare expenditures make up approximately 18% of the U.S. gross domestic product (GDP) (Cleverley, Song, & Cleverley, 2011)

- The United States leads the world in healthcare costs, and these costs are approximately 50% more than the second closest country

- The annual growth rate of annual healthcare costs in the United States from 2007 to 2012 was 5.5% (Cleverley, Song, & Cleverley, 2011)

- The United States has over 50 million individuals that fail to have healthcare insurance and leads the world in administrative costs and the number of hours spent filling out medical forms (Slavin, 2011)

- The average per capital healthcare expenditure is approximately $7,000, which is 14 times larger than what it was in 1950

- The inflationary rate in healthcare is approximately four times greater over the past decade than in the rest of our economy

- The per capita expenditure is almost double that of which is found in other wealthy nations (Slavin, 2011)

CHAPTER 20

The rate of growth in healthcare as part of the GDP exemplifies how having knowledge of basic economic principles is important for administration.

Economic Resources and Economic Efficiency

There are four types of economic resources of paramount importance:

1. **Land** is distinguishable as being fixed in its supply. It includes surface land, minerals, and other natural resources found in the air, soil, and sea.

2. **Labor** is composed of all human physical and mental abilities and qualities used in production of goods and services.

3. **Capital** includes produced goods (e.g., machines, buildings, computers), which are used for factor inputs for further production.

4. **Entrepreneurial** talent involves human decision-making, risk taking, invention, and ingenuity.

Societies try to solve the economic problem of scarcity by using two techniques: allocative (economic) efficiency and technical efficiency (Rycroft, 1992). *Allocative efficiency* is characteristic of a society using its resources to produce the types and quantities of goods and services that best satisfy the needs of their members. Failing to do so wastes valuable resources that could be used elsewhere (Rycroft, 1992). In other words, society attempts to achieve an optimal standard of production that would best serve the needs of its citizens. Producing commodities that they want and need at the level that is demanded is the goal of allocative efficiency. Allocative efficiency is a basic principle found within business organizations, including healthcare organizations. Healthcare organizations, including hospitals, nursing homes, sub-acute rehabilitation institutes, and clinical settings, have to achieve allocative efficiency to be successful.

Technical efficiency exists when society is able to produce the greatest quantity of goods and services possible from their available resources (Rycroft, 1992). Technical efficiency attempts to optimize a society's ability to produce goods and services according to available resources. To do less would be a failure of their technical ability, and this inefficiency would waste society's resources. Businesses, including hospital and nursing home administrators, have to achieve technical efficiency. In an era of cost containment,

BASIC ECONOMIC PRINCIPLES

achieving technical efficiency is needed for healthcare organizations. Superfluous resources and unused capital is an unproductive waste of resources.

Given that a society has a limited amount of resources, the members of society must make choices between the alternatives that are available to them. This is the concept of *opportunity cost*. Opportunity cost is a central problem that has to be worked out in any society's economic system. Due to the scarcity in resources, individuals, businesses, and governments must choose certain opportunities while foregoing others. This is no different for healthcare organizations. When the healthcare administrator impacts one area, it always comes at a cost. This is the basis of economics. Nothing is free, and there is a cost for all decisions that are made. In other words, the opportunity cost of a choice is the value of the best alternative choice that is sacrificed by members of a society (Rycroft, 1992).

Opportunity cost is central to understanding the dynamics of any society, or any organization's economic life within society. There are very few free goods, and most goods and commodities are scarce, requiring society to decide how to best allocate these resources. Moreover, because every society or business faces economic issues of scarcity, understanding the underlying economic tradeoffs that are part of the economic institution in society is imperative. For example, if a healthcare organization decides to invest more money in capital investments, this leaves less that can be spent on labor. On the personal level, if a person decides to buy a new automobile, they may have to forego buying the new computer they wanted. Therefore, opportunity cost or making choices is central to economic reality.

One way to envision the concept of opportunity cost and how certain choices affect other areas of our lives is to examine a production possibility curve. This curve examines the productive ability of a society between two types of goods and services. It demonstrates what happens when one resource is chosen at the expense of other resources. The diagram below demonstrates a production possibility curve between two randomly chosen products: eggs and butter.

This curve demonstrates that when resources are limited, the production of one commodity will influence the resources available to produce a second product. The following can be determined by reviewing the curve:

CHAPTER 20

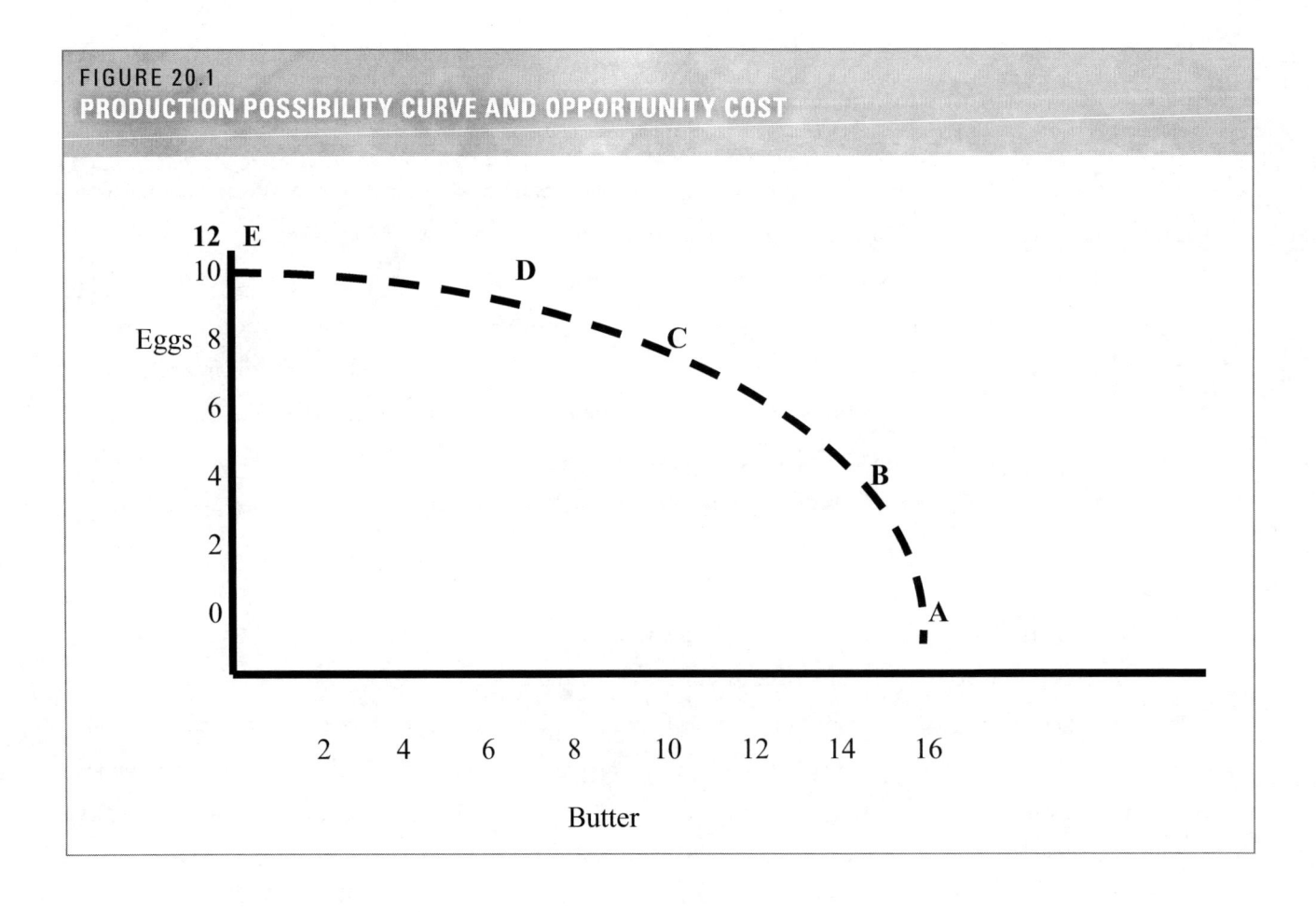

FIGURE 20.1
PRODUCTION POSSIBILITY CURVE AND OPPORTUNITY COST

- At point A, if 16 butters are produced, no resources are available to produce any eggs.

- At point B, if 14 butters are produced, there are enough resources left to produce approximately 4 eggs.

- At point C, if 10 butters are produced, there are enough resources left to produce 8 eggs.

- At point D, if 8 butters are produced, there are enough resources left to produce 10 eggs.

- At point E, if one uses all their resources to produce 12 eggs, no butter can be produced.

Although this is a hypothetical example based on two unrelated commodities, the essence of the example is that on the basis of opportunity cost, resources are limited. Since there is always a scarcity of resources, making a choice in one area will have an economic impact on choices made in other areas. This is a central economic concern in any area of healthcare management.

BASIC ECONOMIC PRINCIPLES

What the production possibility curve shows and the concept of opportunity cost demonstrates is that there are always tradeoffs that have to be considered on the economic level. It also leads to the concepts of *increasing relative costs* and *diminishing returns*. These are really two separate concepts subsumed under the titles of the law of increasing relative costs and the law of diminishing returns. Let us examine the important concept of the law of increasing relative costs first.

The law of relative costs states that as more of a good or service is produced, the opportunity cost also rises. Notice that this is the relative cost. This means the cost of producing a unit in relation to another unit. For example, going back to the production possibility curve, at point A, when 16 butters were produced, no eggs were produced. However at point B, only 14 butters could be produced when four eggs were produced. At point A, no eggs lead to 16 units of butter. But now there is an increasing relative cost, where at point B, 3.5 units of butter can be produced for every one egg unit. The relative cost increases at point C, where 10 butters and 8 eggs are produced. Now only 1.25 units of butter can be produced for every one egg produced. Notice the increasing relative cost.

The law of relative cost is due to the law of diminishing returns. The law of diminishing returns happens where each additional unit of input adds less and less to total output. Let us use the following arbitrary grouping as an example. Let each number stand for a particular unit of something.

Unit of productivity (workers)	Total output	Marginal output
1	3	3
2	7	4
3	12	5
4	20	8
5	26	6
6	31	5 } Point of diminishing return
7	34	3

In this example, notice what is happening. Total output continues to increase all the way through. With each additional worker, the total output is increased. However, marginal output is key. Marginal output is the increase in output for each additional unit of production (in this case, workers) added. Marginal output continues to increase up to a point. It increases up to four workers. However, now adding the fifth worker is really coming at a greater cost, as each additional unit of input actually leads to a decrease in marginal

CHAPTER 20

output, or a decrease in what each additional unit can produce. At the point of diminishing returns, the company should not be adding any more input due to the increase in relative costs that exist.

What Is the Gross Domestic Product?

Before going further, a very important economic concept should be defined. GDP is the nation's total expenditures on the final goods and services that are produced by the country within a given year. For 2011, the GDP was almost 15 trillion (14.9 trillion). To place this in perspective, in 1929, the GDP was 104 billion dollars for the United States. In 1970, our GDP went over 1 trillion dollars, moving to 2.7 trillion in 1980, 5.8 trillion in 1990, and reaching 9.9 trillion in 2000 (Slavin 2011). As one can see, the U.S. GDP has increased approximately 15 times over the last four decades. It took 41 years, from 1929 to 1970, to go from 100 billion to 1 trillion dollars and from 1970 to 2011, another 41 year period, we went from slightly over one trillion dollars in GDP to almost 15 trillion! The U.S. GDP appears to be growing geometrically without any intent of slowing down.

It was mentioned that health expenditures that currently make up a percentage of the GDP are almost at 18%. In 1960, approximately 5% of the GDP was made up of healthcare expenditures. This totaled approximately 7% in 1970. In 1980, it was still in single digits at approximately 9%. However between 1980 and 1990, healthcare expenditures went past 10%, crossing the 10% mark for the first time in 1982. Over the past three decades, the growth of healthcare expenditures as part of GDP has grown incredibly, with a healthcare inflationary status that is becoming quite troubling.

According to the Centers for Medicare & Medicaid Services, healthcare will make up approximately 19.5% of the GDP by 2017 (KaiserEDU.org). Hospital care and physician clinical services alone account for 51% of the total annual healthcare expenditures that make up the GDP (KaiserEDU.org). Of the almost 18% of healthcare expenditures that make up the GDP, the breakdown of the costs are as follows (KaiserEDU.org):

- 31% is spent on hospital care

- 20% on physician and clinical services

- 10% on retail prescription drugs

- 7% on other professional services

BASIC ECONOMIC PRINCIPLES

- 6% on net cost of health insurance

- 6% on investment

- 5% on nursing home care

- 5% on other health residential personal care

- 3% for home healthcare

- The remaining amount was for residual government and retail expenses

So one may ask, what makes up the concept of the GDP? Healthcare administrators are not responsible for determining the GDP—that is a task relegated to the economists—but having a basic understanding of what the GDP is, how it plays an important role in explaining healthcare expenditures, as well as how GDP places healthcare costs into a larger context for society is important for administrators. The equation to determine the GDP is as follows:

$$GDP = C + I + G + X_n$$

What this equation states is that the gross domestic product is equal to the total expenditures on personal consumption, investment, government spending, and net exports. Each one can be further defined as such:

- Personal consumption (C). This is the total amount spent by households over a given year. This is the largest part of the gross domestic product, accounting for approximately 70% of the GDP (Slavin, 2011).

- Investment (I). This includes capital goods, new plant expenditures, equipment, and additional business inventor.

- Government spending (G). This includes all government purchases, including federal, state, and local government, of goods and services.

- Net Exports (Xn). Imports are included under this function but are subtracted to represent our total product of goods and services that have net export value in a given year.

CHAPTER 20

Therefore, hypothetically, if you had 5 trillion in consumption, 2 trillion in investment, 3 trillion in government spending, 2 trillion in exports, and 1 trillion in imports, we would have the following:

5 trillion (C) + 2 trillion (I) + 3 trillion (G) + 1 trillion (Xn) = 11 trillion GDP

Inflation, Unemployment, and Economic Growth

Inflation, unemployment, and economic growth are paramount concerns in any economic system, but the importance of these concepts, mixed with their potential volatility, is especially important for the market economy. Although these three concepts are separate features of economic life, they are often related. How are these factors relevant to a healthcare administrator? First, healthcare is part of the larger economic system of our country. Second, at almost 18% of the GDP, it makes a significant contribution to our total economic landscape. Finally, the economics of healthcare are not insulated from the larger economic environment, and the larger economic landscape—even that which is not directly part of healthcare—still has an incredible impact on healthcare economics.

Inflation deals with the general increase in the average price of goods and services found in society. Between the years of 1770 and 1940, there were very low rates of inflation in our society, with inflationary years balanced out by deflationary years. However, since the 1940s, inflation has been an important issue to American society and has continued to increase substantially (Slavin, 2011). The value of the dollar has continued to shrink in proportion to the increasing rate of inflation. For example, a dollar as measured on the basis of its 1998 value would have been worth $8.36 in 1946. In 1960, its worth was reduced to $5.51, in 1970, it was reduced further to $4.02. Additionally, an item that cost $1.00 in 1982 would have cost approximately 10 cents in 1913, 18 cents in 1945, and $2.23 in 2010 (The World Almanac, 2012).

Unemployment rates have also been a serious concern in our society, especially since approximately 2007. *Unemployment* is related to the level of inflation in society. Professor A.W. Phillips, who studied this trend over a number of years, found that there is a trade-off between the rate of inflation in society and the level of unemployment. Although this trade-off is not perfectly predictable, there does appear to be an inverse relationship between inflation and unemployment. This means that when inflation increases, the level of unemployment decreases. Conversely, when prices decrease, the general rate of unemployment tends to increase. This relationship is known as the Phillips curve.

Economic policy is often concerned about this trade-off and to what level they should control inflation to produce an unemployment rate that is healthy for our society's economic life. However, again, what level

BASIC ECONOMIC PRINCIPLES

of inflation is optimal for society, or even if inflation to any appreciable level is healthy for society is not consensually agreed upon in the economic community. Inflation within the healthcare sector has been one of the highest in the overall economy. Inflationary costs have become an endemic issue and prominent concern for our healthcare industry and the health of our healthcare system.

Returning back to the discussion of the Phillips curve, it can be stated that it does not always follow its predicted path. During periods of stagflation, a condition in which there is both high unemployment and high inflation such as was experienced by our country from 1979 to 1981, the Phillips curve shows this vulnerability. In this example, the Phillips curve failed to demonstrate any predictive validity toward solving this problem or illuminating reasons for this particular economic downturn. Nevertheless, the Phillips curve does demonstrate a fairly consistent association between inflation and unemployment and can be used as a rough benchmark to understand the interaction between inflation and unemployment. The following diagram illustrates what is known as the Phillips curve. Notice the inverse relationship between the rate of inflation and unemployment.

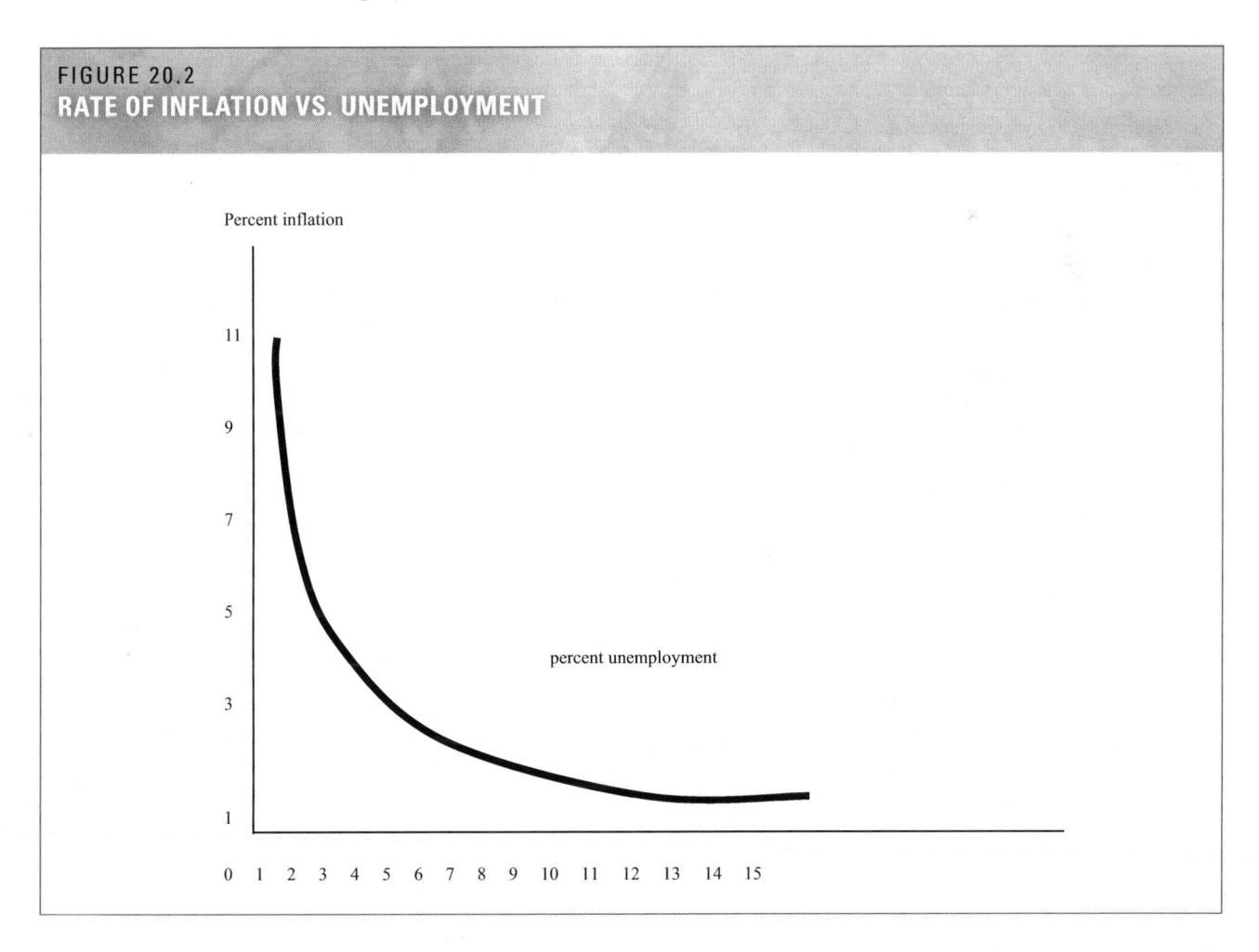

FIGURE 20.2
RATE OF INFLATION VS. UNEMPLOYMENT

CHAPTER 20

Another important consideration is the relationship between unemployment and economic growth. Arthur Okun studied this phenomenon just as Phillips did. Okun was a highly influential Yale economist and one of the most influential economic advisors to Presidents Kennedy and Johnson. Similar to the finding of Phillips, Okun found that economic growth was inversely related to unemployment. As economic growth increased, rates of unemployment in society decreased. In his historical analysis of the relationship between these two variables, he found that for every 2.2% of real growth in the GDP, the unemployment rate subsequently fell by 1%. This became known as Okun's Law. This follows the thinking of Phillips, because as aggregate demand increases in society, the price level will rise, followed by an increase in the GDP, which will subsequently lead to a fall in the unemployment rate.

Supply and Demand in the Market Economy

There are two major economic forms in the contemporary world: the market economy and the centrally regulated economy. In the *market economy*, the state does not actively regulate the economic activities of the society, believing that market forces will direct the economy in the right direction. However, market economies are usually not pure in form; therefore, there is often varying degrees of government regulation mixed with varying degrees of economic activity directed by the forces of supply and demand. Our economy is predominately driven by market forces, but government intervention through Medicare and Medicaid forms of reimbursement demonstrate the mixed nature of our economic world. In the *centrally regulated economies*, the state plays the most prominent role in the economic activities of society, including determining the supply and demand that will exist. In reality, there is no pure market or centrally regulated economy, and most contemporary societies exhibit features of both, although one form will usually predominate.

Capitalism is an economic system based mainly on the market theory. It refers to a system founded on the belief in private property (privatization), competition, and the pursuit of profit without government interference. Adam Smith promoted the original tenets of capitalism, stating that the combination of private property and pursuit of profit would be beneficial to society. Smith stated that competition would motivate capitalists to make higher quality goods and services for the consumer as well as promote a more efficient use of resources to help reduce cost. Smith believed that the economy should be left alone and that the "invisible hand" of the market economy should direct the economic behavior of society. Capitalism is quite dependent on the invisible forces of supply and demand being determined by a freely interacting and unrestricted market sector. Additionally, property ownership belongs to private individuals and not to the state. The theory behind private property ownership is based on the belief that people have inalienable

BASIC ECONOMIC PRINCIPLES

rights to own and control their own property, and private property will make and encourage the pursuit of profit possible. Although no pure system of capitalism exists, societies that have predominately capitalistic economic systems strongly pay attention to the forces of supply and demand that are usually determined by consumer wants and needs. The supply and demand for a product will influence the price of a commodity or a service, such as healthcare. The capitalistic market systems seek to achieve equilibrium, where supply is equal to demand. However, the free movement of supply and demand settling at a level of equilibrium is not always as easy and free-moving as Adam Smith had supposed. The following graph illustrates this market process.

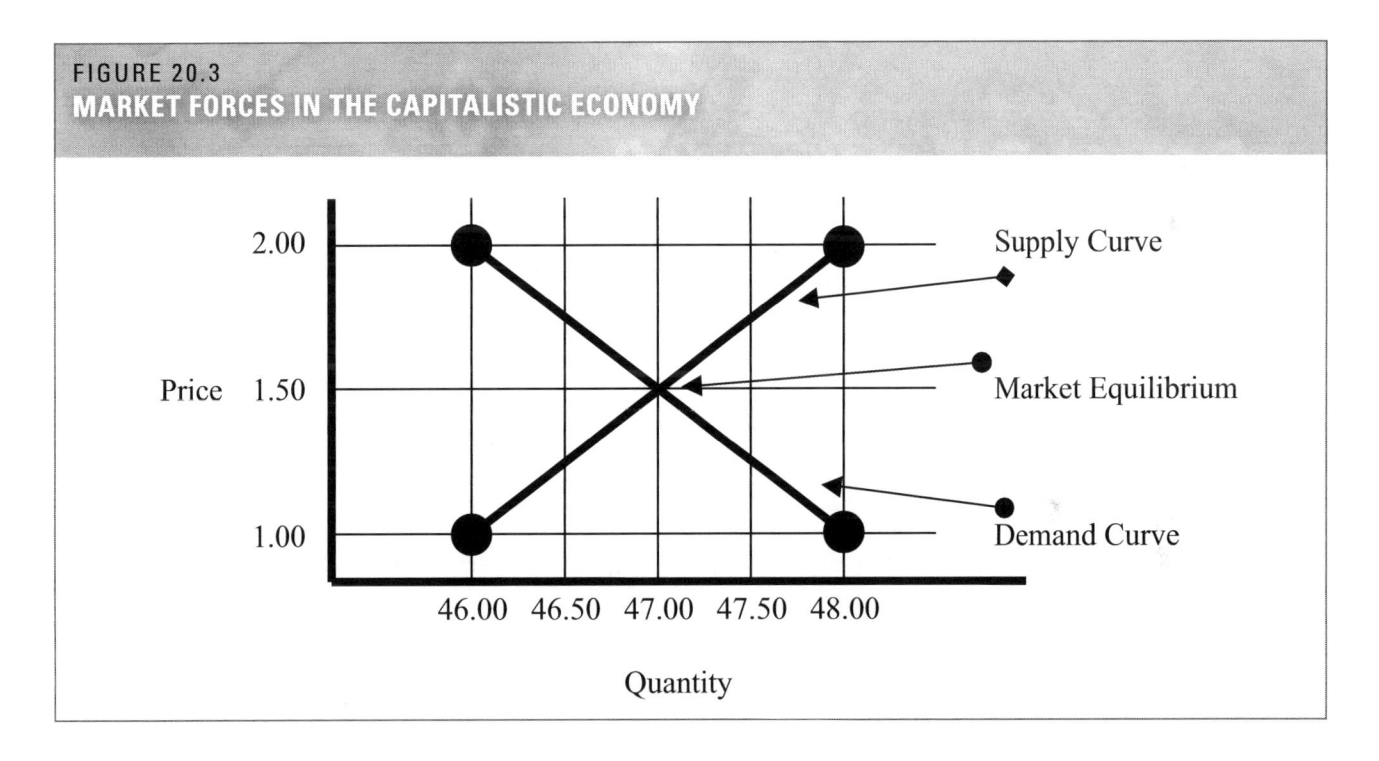

FIGURE 20.3
MARKET FORCES IN THE CAPITALISTIC ECONOMY

This graph demonstrates that as supply increases, so does price. Conversely, the demand curve demonstrates that demand is inversely related to prices—as demand increases, price decreases and vice versa. As the forces of supply and demand fluctuate in the market economy, eventually an equilibrium price will be established where supply of particular goods and services equals the demand for them. In this example, equilibrium is reached when the quantity supplied (47.00) equaled the price that people were willing and able to pay for the particular commodity ($1.50).

As mentioned, if left alone, the forces of supply and demand supposedly achieve equilibrium. Using the same diagram as described above, we can see how this works. By looking at supply in the example, what happens when supply decreases and then when supply is increased?

CHAPTER 20

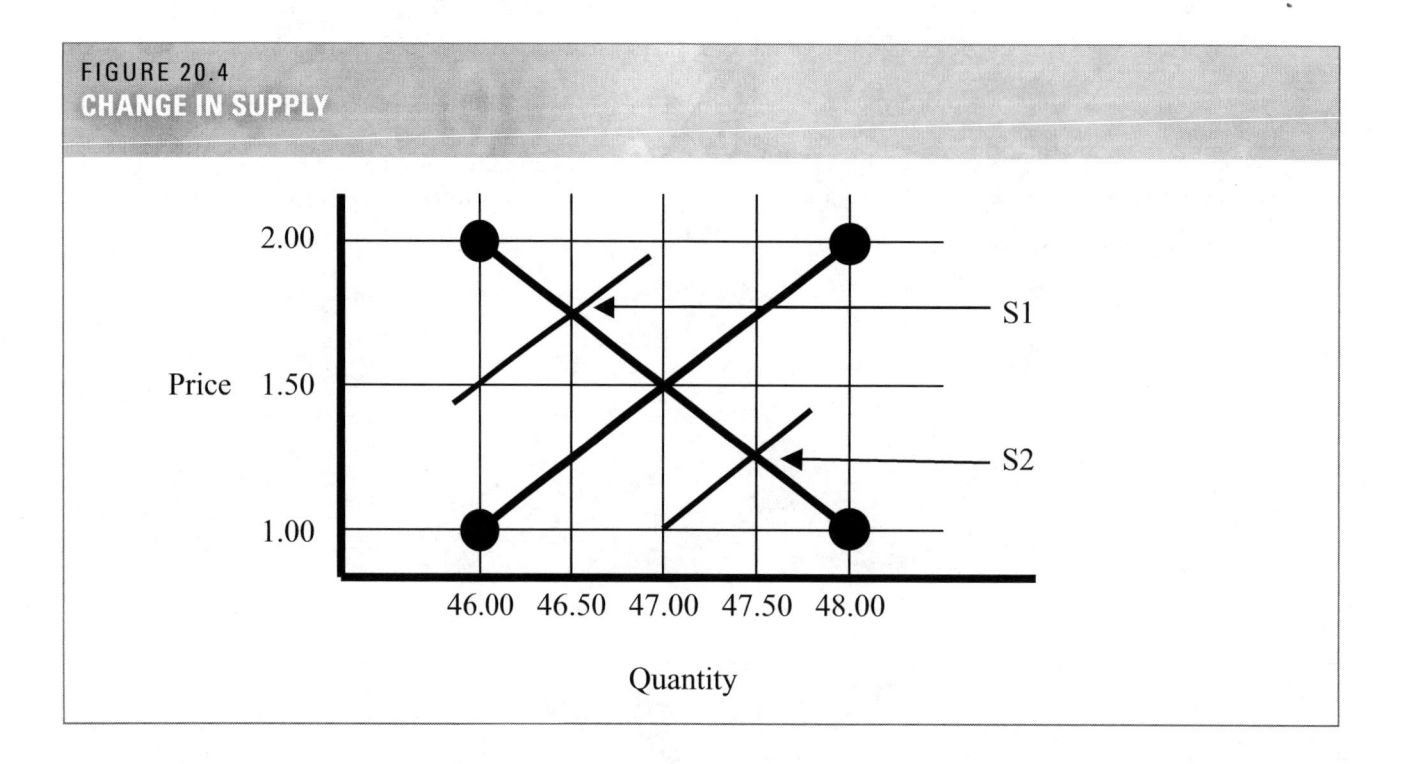

FIGURE 20.4
CHANGE IN SUPPLY

Remember that the original equilibrium was at a quantity of 47 and a price of $1.50. This is noted by the larger supply and demand curve crossing at that point. If the supply is reduced, as denoted by S1, the supply curve shifts upward and to the left. S1, the new supply curve, now crosses the demand curve at approximately $1.75 and at a quantity at 46.50. If the supply is increased, the curve shifts downward and to the right. Now look at the new equilibrium. The quantity is 47.50 and the price is approximately $1.25.

In the previously described scenario, consider what happens to the quantity as it relates to the price, especially as it relates to demand. In S1, when the supply is reduced, costs increase and quantity decreases. The scarcity of the product increased the price. Conversely, in S2, the supply became more available, leading to more quantity offered and subsequently a decrease in price. The cost of resources, changes in the technology available, price expectations for particular goods and services, as well as unexpected events (e.g., unexpected petroleum embargos) can affect the supply and ultimately the equilibrium within the market economy. Supplies of certain healthcare services are also influenced by these market forces.

Now take a look at the change in the demand curve using the diagram below. This is the same analogy as supply, only it has been labeled as D1 and D2. As in the earlier example, the original equilibrium was at a quantity of 47.00 and a price of $1.50. In D1, demand increases, shifting the curve upward and to the right. Therefore, as the demand for a good or service increases, so does the quantity offered and the price. The new equilibrium is at the quantity of 47.00 and the price of $1.75.

BASIC ECONOMIC PRINCIPLES

However, as fewer people want a particular good or service, notice what happens—demand decreases. With decreased demand, the price also decreases. This is seen by a downward left shift in the demand curve. Subsequently, a new market equilibrium has been established—at a quantity of 46.50 and a price of $1.25.

There are a number of things that can lead to a change in demand. For example, consumer tastes can change and with it demand for a good or service. Changes in income can influence demand, such as the recent downturn in the economy, which has led to many individuals losing their jobs and with it losing their health insurance and having less income to seek healthcare services. Furthermore, prices of alternative goods and services can influence demand, as can price expectations within a given area.

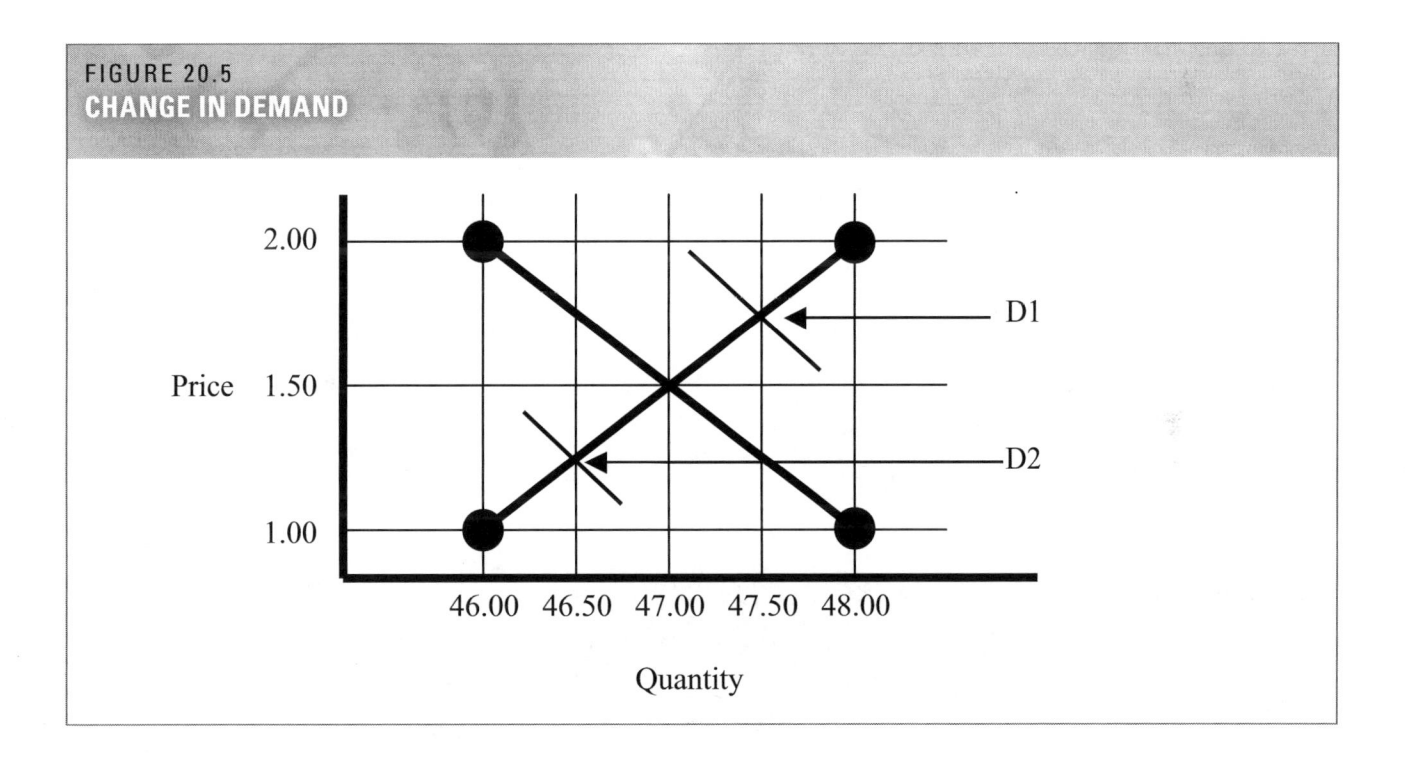

FIGURE 20.5
CHANGE IN DEMAND

Shifts in the Scale of Production

Administrators in any area of business have to consider future levels of operation, and healthcare is no different. Administrators and managers cannot just look at what is currently happening but also must consider the economics of expansion and future growth of the company. This does not mean that the company or healthcare facility will grow, but it often needs to be an economic consideration based on existing viability. Long-term planning is essential for sound administration, and yet the resources that are

CHAPTER 20

available for possible growth are finite. Nevertheless, the business will experience changes in average costs as the size of the company changes. When inputs are changed at the same time and at the same proportion, economists often refer to this as *scales of production.*

Returns to scales of production can exist at three levels: diminishing returns to scale, constant returns to scale, and increasing returns to scale. *Diminishing returns to scale (DRS)* occur when an increase in inputs leads to less than a proportionate increase in outputs. For example, if one additional monetary unit was added, leading to only a marginal increase of only three quarters of additional output, this is considered diminishing returns to scale. With a *constant return to scale (CRS)*, input added is proportional to output achieved. If an administrator doubled the capital enhancement added to the physical therapy unit and realized a doubling in the revenue from physical therapy, a constant return in scale has been achieved. Finally, with *increasing returns to scale (IRS)*, an increase in input leads to more than a proportionate increase in total output. In the example above, if an administrator increased the annual capital enhancement budget for physical therapy by two times and realized revenue that was five times greater, this was two and one half times greater in revenue realization than inputs invested.

Increasing returns to scale often leads to the important concept known as *economies of scale.* A healthcare organization that has realized an economy of scale has increased its efficiency and demonstrates a decrease in average cost as the firm expands. With economies of scale, an increase in output exceeds the level of proportionate input. Furthermore, as quantity increases, average total cost decreases, as demonstrated by the negative slope of the figure below.

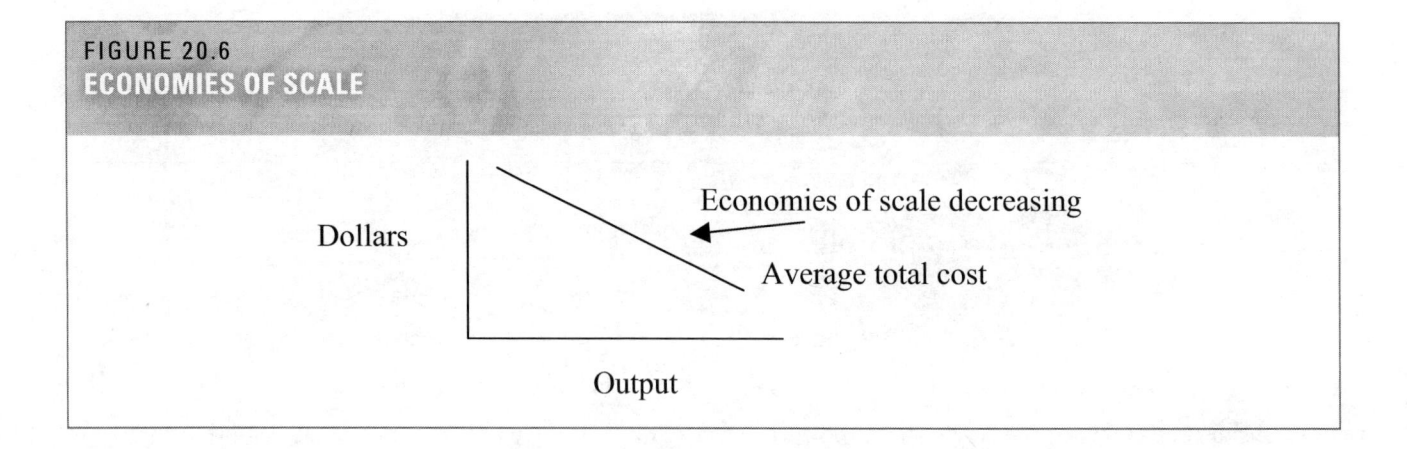

FIGURE 20.6
ECONOMIES OF SCALE

BASIC ECONOMIC PRINCIPLES

Diseconomies of scale is the opposite of economies of scale. This can happen due to poor management or when an organization expands too quickly—a common occurrence in many healthcare facilities today. In this situation, diminishing costs of scale often exist and costs start to rise quickly and at an uncontrolled rate. The figure below demonstrates changes that are brought about by a diseconomy of scale. Notice as unit of outputs increase, so do dollars.

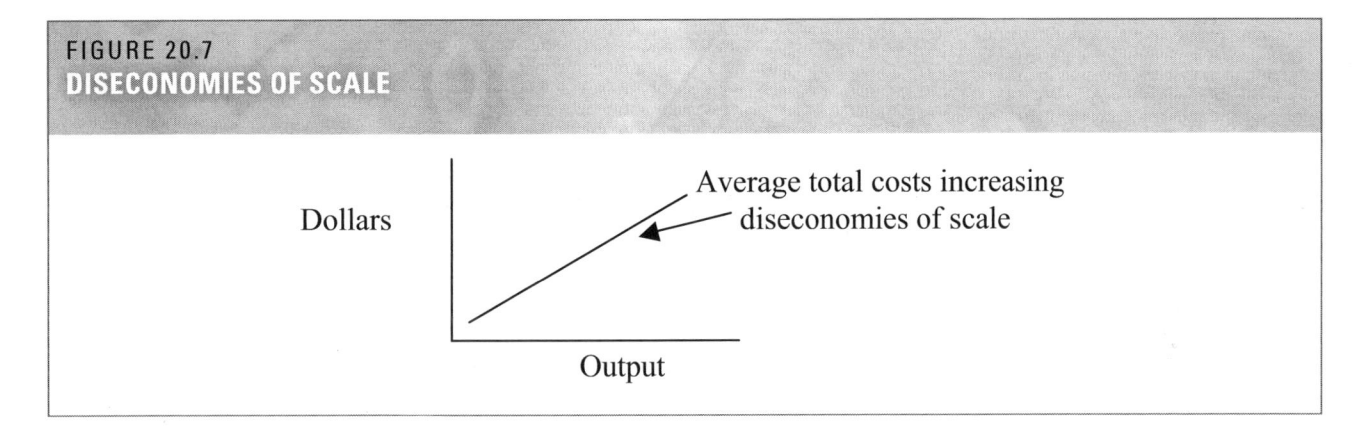

FIGURE 20.7
DISECONOMIES OF SCALE

[Graph showing Dollars on vertical axis and Output on horizontal axis, with an upward-sloping line labeled "Average total costs increasing diseconomies of scale"]

Consumer Behavior and Utility

A basic premise of economics revolves around the concept of self-interest. Individuals are self-interested consumers, and this is viewed as a basic motivational tool for them to consume. Regardless of whether consumption is looking at purchasing an automobile, an ice cream cone, or a healthcare product, the economics of utility for the self-interested consumer is very important. So how does economic theory view consumer behavior and what is utility as a driving force for such behavior?

When utility is spoken about in economics, it is not synonymous with usefulness. Utility is often a subjective concept that is viewed as the satisfaction that the consumer derives from the product. Economic theory states that since money is finite and since consumers are self-interested in spending their money in a manner that provides them with the greatest satisfaction, the need to understand how economic utility is achieved is important toward addressing consumer desiderata. Economics refers to a unit of economic satisfaction as a "util," which is short for utility. Consumer behavior and utility are very important in healthcare consumption.

CHAPTER 20

Economically speaking, the utility of something, or its "util" value, is not constant. It changes. The util of something is usually greatest at the beginning, after which there is a diminishing law of marginal utility. Consider this simple example: You are very hungry and have not eaten in a couple of days. Now you have four sandwiches in front of you. You eat the first sandwich and derive tremendous satisfaction from the experience. You then eat the second sandwich since you are still hungry, but not as hungry as you started. After eating the third sandwich you are full. You decide to eat the fourth sandwich because it is available, but then feel bloated, uncomfortable, and somewhat nauseous from eating too much. The following graph illustrates this example:

Sandwich	Marginal utils	Total utils
First	+100	+100
Second	+50	+150
Third	+10	+160
Fourth	−30	+130

Notice that the greatest utility was achieved after the first sandwich, especially in addressing your hunger. It provided a marginal utility of +100 (the points are just arbitrary to help quantity the description). The consumption of the second sandwich provides less satisfaction or utility at 50 utils. The third sandwich adds another positive 10 utils, but still less positive satisfaction. Then you ate the fourth sandwich when you already were full and it made you ill by being too full. Its marginal utility was −30. Furthermore, look what happens to the total utility with the fourth sandwich—it went from positive 160 down to positive 130. Ideally, you should have stopped eating when your total utility was increasing.

What the earlier graph shows is something referred to as the *Law of Marginal Utility*. Each identical good or service consumed within a given period of time will provide you with less and less satisfaction, as demonstrated by the marginal utils. However, as long as the marginal utility is positive and it does not subtract from the total utility, one can continue to add more units. When the next unit will lead to negative marginal utility and therefore also reduce total utility, there should not be any further consumption. The following figure demonstrates these concepts as economists like to visualize them for the audience:

BASIC ECONOMIC PRINCIPLES

FIGURE 20.8
TOTAL UTILITY

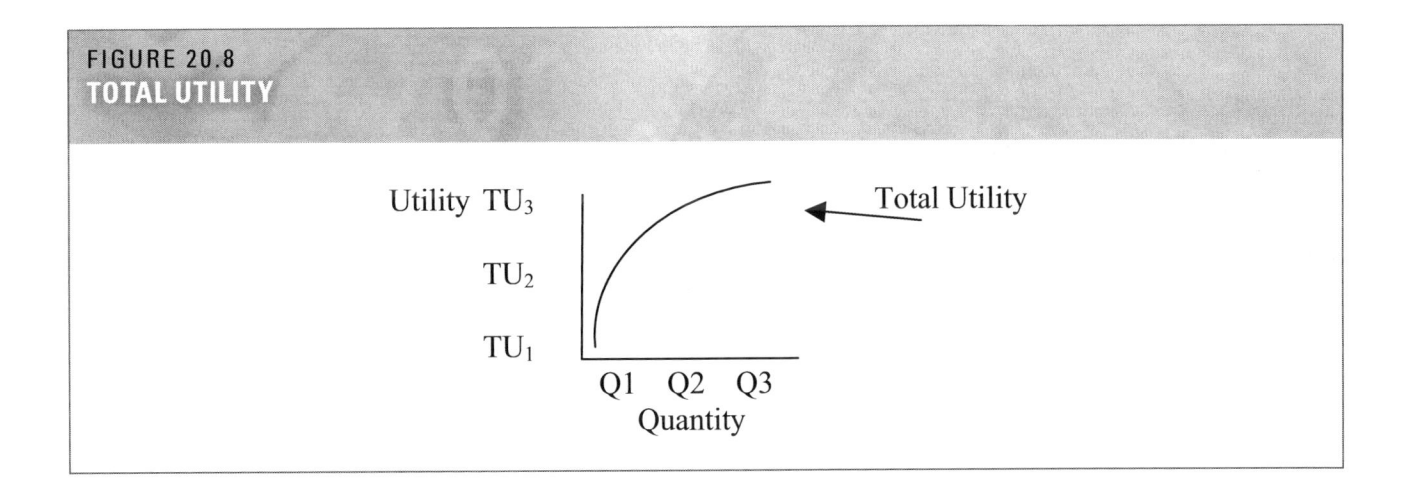

Utility TU$_3$, TU$_2$, TU$_1$ vs. Quantity (Q1, Q2, Q3) — Total Utility curve.

Total utility continues to increase but increases much slower over a period of time. In fact, the velocity of change is quick at first, but within a very short period of time, the *velocity of change* slows quite noticeably. The following figure looks at what happens at marginal utility simultaneously with total utility.

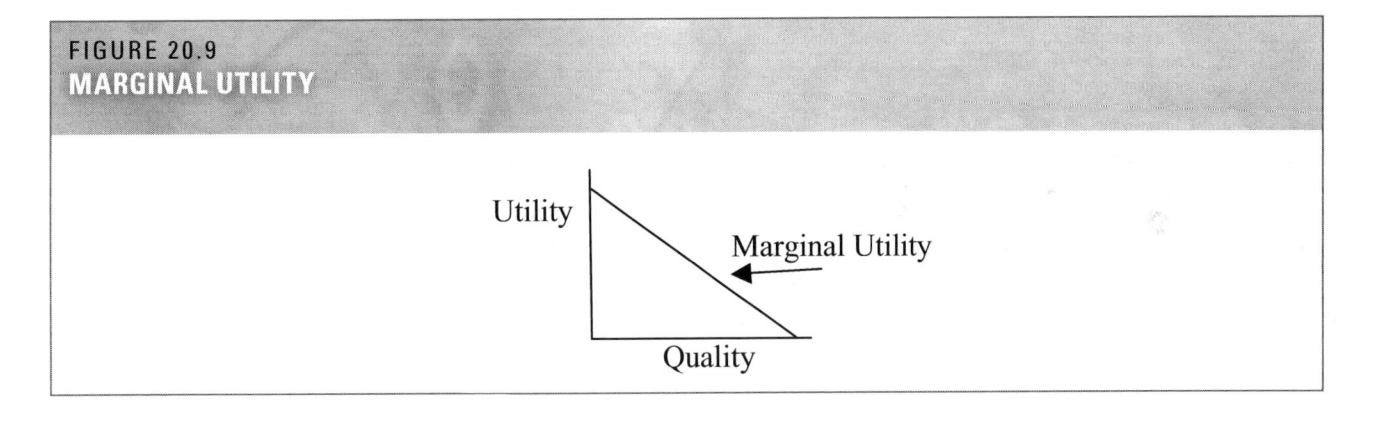

FIGURE 20.9
MARGINAL UTILITY

Utility vs. Quality — Marginal Utility curve.

Recall that total utility was increasing, although at an increasingly slower velocity. Simultaneously, marginal utility is decreasing. Notice also the sharply declining slope of marginal utility. As was mentioned above, marginal utility decreases very quickly, with the greatest satisfaction being derived from the first unit, and, thereafter, it decreases quite precipitously.

Consider another economic principle as it relates to marginal utility. As consumption increases, total utility increases, but marginal utility decreases. This was witnessed in the previously described example.

Finance, Budgeting & Quantitative Analysis: A Primer for Nursing Home Administrators

CHAPTER 20

FIGURE 20.10
MAXIMUM TOTAL UTILITY

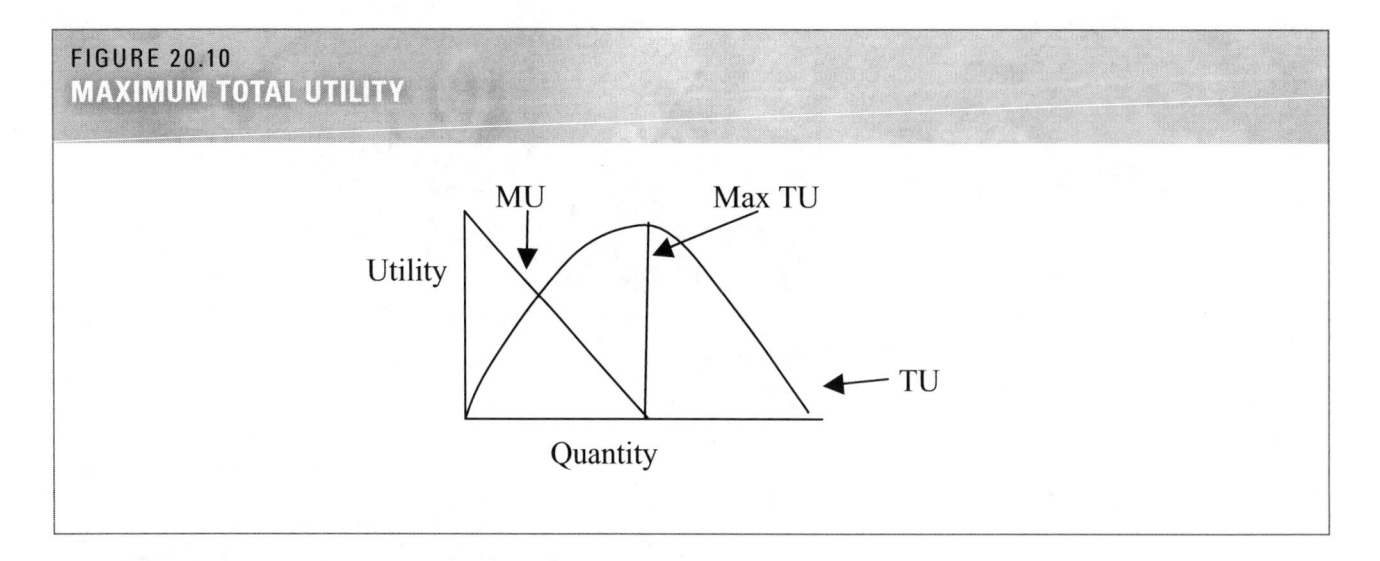

But also consistent with this principle, there is a maximum total utility. This can be diagrammed as follows:

As is evident by this figure, the marginal utility slope demonstrates a very quick, precipitous decline. As the curve continues to the right, its total utility continues to increase, but maximum total utility exists where marginal utility and total utility equal zero. This is where no additional units could be added without the marginal utility becoming negative. The basic economic law here is as follows:

- Marginal utility > 0; this leads approximately to ↑ in TU

- Marginal utility < 0; this leads approximately to ↓ in TU

How Income and Substitution Effects Influence Consumer Behavior

Consumer behavior is often influenced by income and substitute goods or services that are available. Healthcare administrators even witness these effects in attempting to manage costs. For example, many generic medications are substituted for other medications or brand names to assist with cost control. If we hold real income constant while substitute products or services become available, leading to decreased prices, the substitute product will likely be chosen. Consumers do this quite frequently in society. However, management decisions are often based on the substitution effect as well. This is especially important in considering the need to address costs and maintain cost control. As mentioned, pharmaceutical costs are great, and when generic or less expensive substitutes become available, consumers will often choose the cheaper substitute.

BASIC ECONOMIC PRINCIPLES

As an administrator, you purchase product A for $20 per unit and product B for $10 per unit. Then the price of product A decreases to $15 per unit. Given that your income has remained constant, what has happened? The price change of the one good or service causes your real income to increase. Since the price of product A decreased by $5 per unit, you now have that much more income to spend. You now have more purchasing power to spend, since you have more money to use due to price decrease.

Price Elasticity of Supply and Demand

Prices play a role in all phases of the economy. Consumer behavior is often shaped by price and by the supply and demand related to price changes. Many areas of healthcare demonstrate considerable inelasticity, such as necessary care. However, managers often face choices they have to make as consumers of resources for their companies.

Elasticity of demand is based on how responsive consumers are to a change in price. If consumers respond to a change in price as it relates to products or services, this is referred to as elasticity in consumer demand. If price changes and the demand for a product or service does not change, this is referred to as inelasticity of demand. An example of this is a nursing home whose private pay rates for respite care may be lower than the competing nursing homes in the area, leading to individuals to choose this nursing home over their competitors.

Price elasticity of demand is often calculated as follows:

$$\text{Price Elasticity of Demand} = \frac{\text{Percent change in quantity demanded}}{\text{Percent change in price}}$$

Elasticity of demand can be determined as such.

If price changes by 1% and change in quantity demanded is greater than 1%, *elasticity of demand* exists. Elasticity is >1. There is an inverse relationship between price and total revenue. Subsequently, if price increases, total revenue decreases. However, if price decreases, total revenue increases.

CHAPTER 20

If price changes by 1% and change in quantity demanded is less than 1%, *inelasticity of demand* exists. Elasticity is <1. There is a direct relationship between price and total revenue. In this case, if price increases, total revenue increases as well. Conversely, if price decreases, total revenue decreases.

If price changes by 1% and change in quantity demanded equals 1%, this is referred to as *unitary elasticity*. Elasticity = 1. If price either increases or decreases, total revenue remains constant.

Supply can also be examined on the basis of its elasticity. As demand is responsive to price, supply also has a level of responsiveness that can be measured. The elasticity of supply measures the responsiveness of suppliers to changes in prices. Healthcare managers do not only measure demand, but much of their oversight is managing the provision and supply of particular services. Furthermore, they also deal with suppliers that provide services that are necessary to their organizations that they demand. Consistent with the economic laws of supply, as price increases, so will the quantity supplied. For example, a long-term care facility decides to also offer community rehabilitative and exercise therapy services. As price increases, so does the quantity or amount of services in this area offered. Measuring the elasticity of supply for this service and others like it would follow rules similar to those delineated for elasticity of demand. The rules for determining elasticity of supply are as follows:

- If a price changes by 1% and this leads to a greater than 1% change in quantity supplied, supply elasticity exists. P Δ of 1% → >1% Δ Q.

- If a price change of 1% leads to a less than 1% change in quantity supplied, an inelasticity of supply exists. P Δ of 1% → <1% Δ Q.

- Finally, if a 1% change in price leads to a 1% change in quantity, supply is unitary.
  P Δ of 1% → = 1% Δ Q.

Marginal Analysis

Many of the earlier examples include some marginal analysis. However, it is an important business decision-making tool that should be considered separately. Many decisions are made at the margins, meaning that the marginal analysis of an additional unit plays a very fundamental role in managerial decisions. What this means and what marginal analysis addresses is the benefits or costs incurred by adding one additional unit of input of a good or service. Net benefits are the ultimate goal and are defined as the total benefits minus total costs. Wessel states the following are key components of marginal analysis (Wessel, 1987, p. 9):

BASIC ECONOMIC PRINCIPLES

1. Control variables need to be identified—the control variable is the variable that is under consideration to see whether it should be undertaken based on examination of the marginal benefits exceeding or failing to exceed marginal costs

2. Determine what increase in total benefits would incur if one more unit (marginal benefit of one additional unit) of the control variable is added

3. Determine what increase in total costs would incur if one more unit (marginal cost of one additional unit) of the control variable is added

4. If the marginal benefit ≥ the marginal cost, the additional unit should be added

5. If the marginal benefit < the marginal cost, the additional unit should not be added

6. An increase in marginal benefits will increase total benefits

7. An increase in marginal costs will increase total costs

8. A change in net benefits is equal to marginal benefits minus marginal costs

Let us examine this concept through the use of the following example. The physical and occupational therapy department have weekly labor costs/expenses of $17,000 and total revenue of $40,000. The department would like to add one additional therapist. This would increase the labor expense to $18,300 and increase the average total revenue to $41,000. Should adding an additional worker be added? On the basis of the marginal analysis, the answer is no. This is because the marginal cost (MC) of adding one additional worker would be $1,300. However, the marginal benefit through additional revenue (more specifically referred to economically as marginal revenue or MC) incurred would be $1,000 (going from a weekly average of $40,000 to $41,000). Therefore, the marginal cost of adding one additional unit (determining whether to add an additional worker is the control variable) exceeds the marginal benefit (revenue) by $300.

Now, consider a different scenario. Using the same numbers as mentioned above, with a weekly labor cost of $17,000 and a weekly average revenue of $40,000, what would happen if adding one new worker would increase the labor expense to $18,300 and now increase the average total weekly revenue to $41,300.

CHAPTER 20

Adding one new worker would lead to a marginal cost of $1,300. Additionally weekly average revenue would be increased to $41,300. Therefore, there is a marginal benefit of $1,300. In this case the marginal cost (MC) = marginal revenue (MR). The decision now would be to hire the one additional worker. Why? As the rule above states, *if the marginal benefit ≥ the marginal cost, the additional unit should be added.* In this scenario, since the marginal costs were $1,300, this equaled the marginal benefit of $1,300, and consistent with the rule for marginal analysis, anything greater than or equal to should lead to the addition of the unit under consideration.

Total Revenue and Costs and Marginal Revenue and Costs

To understand marginal analysis, one needs to not only address marginal revenue and marginal cost but also demonstrate how these factors relate to total revenue and total costs. Profit for any business is based on total revenue exceeding total costs. Therefore, profit quite simply is as follows:

$$\text{Profit} = \text{Total Revenue} - \text{Total Costs}$$

Diagrammatically, we can demonstrate how total revenue and total costs exist and where profit is maximized. The figure below demonstrates TR and TC.

The previous figure shows that the total revenue (TR) line is the straight line with a linear slope. The total cost curve (TC) starts out moving upward above TR. At this point, an economic loss exists. At point (A), TR = TC, and this is referred to as the break-even point for the business. Then the TC curve goes down and it drops considerably below the TR. The points marked as B and C demonstrate the greatest difference between TR and TC. This is the point where profit is maximized. Then the TC curve starts to move back upward, going to point D, which is again where TR = TC and becomes another break-even point.

Now it is important to consider how marginal revenue (MR) and marginal costs (MC) are related to total revenue and total costs. The slope of the total revenue curve is equal to marginal revenue (MR), and the slope of the total cost curve is equal to marginal cost (MC) (Fogiel 1989). Given this, profit maximization is equal to the point where total revenue is equal to total costs, or MR = MC. Let us take a look at the interaction between MR and MC and how it relates to profit maximization.

BASIC ECONOMIC PRINCIPLES

FIGURE 20.11
TOTAL REVENUE AND TOTAL COST

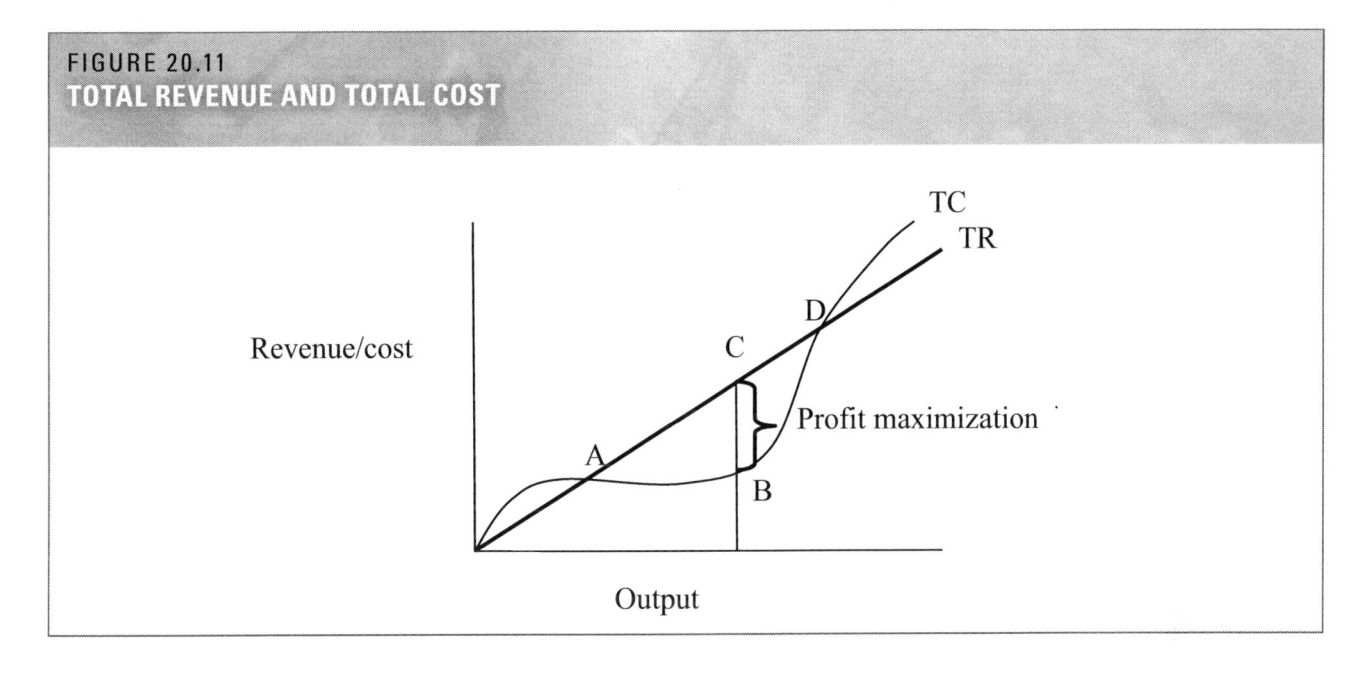

In Q1, notice that MR considerably exceeds MC for the business. This means that additional units can be added since the business still is not producing at profit maximization. However, as more units are added, the MC curve moves upward and crosses the MR curve at Q2. When MR is equal to MC at Q2, profit maximization now exists. This is also where total revenue is at its greatest point of maximization in relation to total cost, as evidenced by the previous figure. Therefore, at MR = MC, any additional units will not incur any greater profit maximization but will incur only increasing amounts of marginal costs. As the MC curve goes above the MR curve, as demonstrated by Q3, MC is now greater than MR. To move back toward profit maximization, the firm would have to decrease its marginal costs, which would entail reducing its outputs and thereby shifting Q3 leftward and back toward Q2.

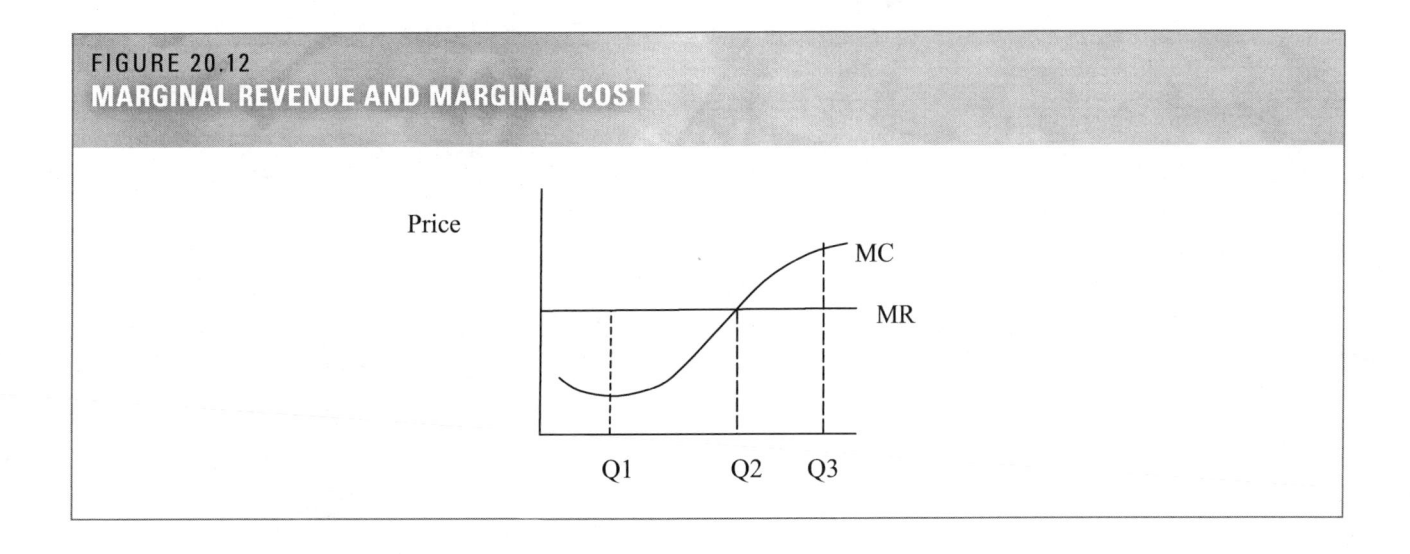

FIGURE 20.12
MARGINAL REVENUE AND MARGINAL COST

References and Suggested Readings

1. Allan, James. 1997. Nursing Home Administration. New York: Springer Publishing Company.

2. Babbie, Earl. 1998. The Practice of Social Research, Eighth Edition. Belmont, CA: Wadsworth Publishing.

3. Becker, Howard. 1998. Tricks of the Trade. Chicago: The University of Chicago Press.

4. Berg, Bruce. 1995. Qualitative Research Methods for the Social Sciences. Needham Heights, MA: Allyn and Bacon Publishing.

5. Boas, Franz. 1943. "Recent Anthropology." *Science* 98: 311–314, 334–337.

6. Boslaugh, S., Watters, P. A. 2008. Statistics in a nutshell. Sebastopol, CA: O'Reily Media, Inc.

7. Britt, David. 1997. A Conceptual Introduction to Modeling—Qualitative and Quantitative Perspectives. Mahwah, NJ: Lawrence Erlbaum Associates, Publishers.

8. The Centers for Medicare & Medicaid Services. National Health Expenditure Data. *www.cms.gov/Research-Statistics-Data-and-Systems/Statistics-Trends-and-Reports/NationalHealthExpendData/index.html?redirect=/NationalHealthExpendData/25_NHE_Fact_Sheet.asp.*

9. The Centers for Medicare & Medicaid Services. Therapy Cap Fact Sheet. *www.cms.gov/Research-Statistics-Data-and-Systems/Monitoring-Programs/Medical-Review/Downloads/TherapyCapFactSheet.pdf.*

REFERENCES AND SUGGESTED READINGS

10. Cleverley, W. O., Song, P. H., Cleverley, J. O. 2011. Essentials of Health Care Finance. Sudbury, MA: Jones & Bartlett Learning.

11. Cockerham, William. 2004. Medical Sociology. Upper Saddle River, NJ: Prentice-Hall Publishing Company.

12. Davis, Winborn, Haacker, Robert, Townsend, Joseph. 2002. The Principles of Health Care Administration. Bossier City, LA: Professional Printing & Publishing, Inc.

13. Denzin, Norman. 1978. The Research Act. New York: McGraw-Hill.

14. Geertz, Clifford. 1973. "Thick Description: Toward an Interpretive Theory of Culture." In The Interpretation of Culture, C. Geertz (Ed). New York: Basic Books.

15. Gill, James O. 1992. Financial Analysis—The Next Step. Los Altos, CA: Crisp Publications, Inc.

16. Habermas, Jurgen. 1970. Knowledge and Human Interest. Trans. by J. Shapiro. London: Heinemann Press.

17. Hollis, Martin. 1996. "Philosophy of Social Science." In The Blackwell Companion to Philosophy, Nicholas Bunnin and E.P. Tsui-James (Eds). Cambridge, MA: Blackwell Publishers, Inc.

18. Humphreys, Laud. 1970. Tearoom Trade: Impersonal Sex in Public Places. Chicago: Aldine Publishers.

19. KaiserEDU.org. U.S. Health Care Costs. *www.kaiseredu.org/Issue-Modules/US-Health-Care-Costs/Background-Brief.aspx#How%20is%20the%20U.S.%20health%20care%20dollar%20spent?*

20. Kuhn, Thomas S. 1970. The Structure of Scientific Revolutions. Chicago: University of Chicago Press.

21. *www.ltc-resources.com*. This website is for both providers and consumers dealing with Medicare benefits for skilled nursing facilities.

REFERENCES AND SUGGESTED READINGS

22. Lindesmith, Alfred. 1947. Opiate Addiction. Bloomington, IN: Principia Press.

23. Lundberg, George. 1964. Foundations of Sociology. New York: David McKay Company, Inc.

24. Medicare.gov. *www.medicare.gov/your-medicare-costs/costs-at-a-glance/costs-at-glance.html*.

25. Moorhead, G., Griffin, R. W. 2004. Organizational Behavior: Managing People and Organizations. Boston: Houghton Mifflin.

26. Mose, Arlene, Jackoson, John, Downs, Gary. 1997. Day-to-Day Business Accounting. Paramus, NJ: Prentice Hall Publishing Company.

27. Neuman, W. Lawrence. 2000. Social Research Methods—Qualitative and Quantitative Approaches. Needham Heights, MA: Allyn and Bacon Publishing.

28. Phillips, John L. 1992. How to Think About Statistics, Revised Edition. New York: W.H. Freeman and Company.

29. Pelto, Pertti J., Pelto, Gretel. 1978. Anthropological Research—The Structure of Inquiry. New York: Cambridge University Press.

30. Pike, Kenneth. 1954. Language in Relation to a Unified Theory of the Structure of Human Behavior, Volume 1. CA: Summer Institute of Linguistics.

31. Plous, Scott. 1993. The Psychology of Judgment and Decision Making. New York: McGraw-Hill.

32. Popper, Karl. 1959. The Logic of Scientific Discovery. London: Hutchinson.

33. Rajagopalan, N., Rasheed, A. M. A., Datta, D. K. 1993. "Strategic Decision Processes: Critical Review and Future Directions." Journal of Management 19(2): 349–384.

34. Rotter, Julian. 1966. "Generalized Expectancies for Internal Versus External Control of Reinforcement." Psychological Monographs 80(1):1–28.

REFERENCES AND SUGGESTED READINGS

35. Rycroft, R. S. 1992. The Essential of Macroeconomics. Research and Education Association. Piscataway, NJ.

36. Schwartz, Howard, Jacobs, Jerry. 1979. Qualitative Sociology: A Method to the Madness. New York: Free Press.

37. Seidel, Lee, Gorsky, R., Lewis, J. 1995. Applied Quantitative Methods for Health Services Management. Baltimore: Health Professionals Press.

38. Silbiger, Steven. 1993. The Ten-Day MBA. New York: William Morrow and Company, Inc.

39. Slavin, S. L. 2011. Economics. New York: McGraw-Hill Irwin.

40. Tuller, Lawrence. 1997. Finance for Non-Financial Managers and Small Business Owners. Holbrook, MA: Adams Media Corporation.

41. United States Department of Labor-Bureau of Labor Statistics, *www.bls.gov/lpc/faqs.htm#P03*.

42. Warren, C. S. 2011. Survey of Accounting. Mason, OH: South-Western Cengage Learning.

43. Wessel, W. J. 1987. Economics. New York, NY: Barron Business Review Series.

44. Weitz, Rose. 2006. The Sociology of Health, Illness, and Healthcare—A Critical Approach. Belmont, CA: Wadsworth Publishing Company.

45. Welch, S., Comer, J. C. 1983. Quantitative Methods for Public Administration. Homewood, Ill: Dorsey Press.